FUNGAL INFECTIONS OF THE SKIN, HAIR AND NAILS

A CD-ROM containing the illustrations from this book is in production.

FUNGAL INFECTIONS

OF THE SKIN, HAIR

AND NAILS

Raimo E Suhonen
Rodney P R Dawber
David H Ellis

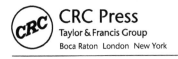

CRC Press

Taylor & Francis Group
Boca Raton London New York

CRC Press is an imprint of the
Taylor & Francis Group, an **informa** business

CRC Press
Taylor & Francis Group
6000 Broken Sound Parkway NW, Suite 300
Boca Raton, FL 33487-2742

First issued in paperback 2019

© 1999 by Taylor & Francis Group, LLC
CRC Press is an imprint of Taylor & Francis Group, an Informa business

No claim to original U.S. Government works

ISBN-13: 978-1-85317-589-3 (hbk)
ISBN-13: 978-0-367-39973-3 (pbk)

Visit the Taylor & Francis Web site at
http://www.taylorandfrancis.com

and the CRC Press Web site at
http://www.crcpress.com

CONTENTS

PREFACE

In the field of fungal infections of the skin, hair and nails many books have been written – typically detailed, heavily referenced texts; or in contrast, small and brief pocket books often aimed at clinicians below the experienced dermatological level. Our combined experience covers all aspects of skin mycology from the laboratory to the academic and pragmatic components of patient care.

We believe that this text atlas format will give the clinician in medicine at large more insight into skin, hair and nail mycology from the diagnostic and therapeutic points of view.

RES

RPRD

DHE

1 AETIOLOGY AND LABORATORY DIAGNOSIS

The cutaneous mycoses are superficial fungal infections of the skin, hair or nails. Essentially no living tissue is invaded. However, a variety of pathological changes occur in the host because of the presence of the infectious agent and/or its metabolic products. The principal aetiological agents are as follows: dermatophytic moulds belonging to the genera *Microsporum, Trichophyton* and *Epidermophyton* which cause ringworm or tinea of the scalp, glabrous skin and nails; *Malassezia (Pityrosporon) furfur*, a lipophilic yeast responsible for pityriasis versicolor, follicular pityriasis, seborrhoeic dermatitis and dandruff; and *Candida albicans* and related species, which cause candidiasis of skin, mucous membrane and nails; the latter may also colonise many moist skin eruptions without being causative.

In world terms, fungal infections of the skin, hair and nails are some of the commonest infections in humanity. The development of very active and successful antifungal drugs in recent years has greatly increased clinical interest in these particular infective agents. The advent of very potent immunosuppressive drugs for a variety of diseases (including HIV infection) has also enabled a variety of fungi to penetrate and cause severe superficial and systemic spread that was previously extremely rare.

Aetiological agents

Dermatophytosis (tinea or ringworm) of the scalp, skin and nails

Dermatophytosis of the scalp, glabrous skin and nails is caused by a closely related group of fungi known as dermatophytes which have the ability to utilise keratin as a nutrient source, i.e. they have a unique enzymatic capacity (keratinase). The disease process in dermatophytosis is unique for two reasons: first, no living tissue is invaded – the keratinised stratum corneum, hair or nail is simply colonised. However, the presence of the fungus and its metabolic products typically induces an inflammatory response in the host. The type and severity of the host response are often related to the species and strain of dermatophyte causing the infection. Second, the dermatophytes are the only fungi that have evolved a dependency on human or animal infection for the survival and dissemination of their species. In fact, the common anthropophilic species (Table 1.1) are primarily parasitic on humans. They are unable to colonise other animals and have no other environmental sources. Geophilic species normally inhabit the soil where they are believed to decompose keratinaceous debris. Some species may cause infections in animals and humans following contact with soil. Zoophilic species are primarily parasitic on animals and infections may be transmitted to humans following contact with the animal host (Table 1.1). Zoophilic infections usually evoke a

Table 1.1 Ecology of common dermatophyte species

Species	Natural habitat	Incidence
Epidermophyton floccosum	Humans	Common
Trichophyton rubrum	Humans	Very common
T. mentagrophytes var. interdigitale	Humans	Common
Trichophyton tonsurans	Humans	Common
Trichophyton violaceum	Humans	Less common
Trichophyton concentricum	Humans	Rare*
Trichophyton schoenleinii	Humans	Rare*
Trichophyton soudanense	Humans	Rare*
Microsporum audouinii	Humans	Less common*
Microsporum ferrugineum	Humans	Less common*
T. mentagrophytes var. mentagrophytes	Mice, rodents	Common
Trichophyton equinum	Horses	Rare
Trichophyton verrucosum	Cattle	Rare
T. mentagrophytes var. quinckeanum	Mice, hedgehogs	Rare*
T. mentagrophytes var. erinacei	Cats	Common
Microsporum canis	Soil	Common
Microsporum gypseum	Soil/pigs	Rare
Microsporum nanum	Soil	Rare
Microsporum cookei		

*Geographically restricted.

strong host response on the skin where contact with the infective animal has occurred, i.e. arms, legs, body or face.

Infections by anthropophilic dermatophytes are usually caused by the shedding of skin scales containing viable infectious hyphal elements (arthroconidia) of the fungus. Desquamated skin scales may remain infectious in the environment for months or years. Therefore transmission may take place by indirect contact long after the infective debris has been shed. Substrates, such as carpet and matting that hold skin scales, make excellent vectors. Thus, transmission of such dermatophytes as *Trichophyton rubrum*, *T. mentagrophytes* var. *interdigitale* and *Epidermophyton floccosum* is usually via the feet. In this site infections are often chronic and may remain subclinical for many years only to become apparent when spread to another site, usually the groin or skin. It is important to recognise that the toe web spaces are the major reservoir on the human body for these fungi and therefore it is not practical to treat infections at other sites without concomitant treatment of the toe web spaces. This is essential if 'cure' is to be achieved. It should also be recognised that individuals with chronic or subclinical toe web infections are carriers and are constantly shedding infectious skin scales.

Onychomycosis

Onychomycosis or fungal infection of the nails may be caused by either dermatophyte fungi (tinea unguium) or non-dermatophyte fungi and yeasts. Dermatophytes are the principal pathogens, accounting for 90% of toenail infections and at least 50% of fingernail infections. *Trichophyton rubrum* and *T. mentagrophytes* var. *interdigitale* are the dominant dermatophyte species involved. *Candida* is mainly associated with paronychia that initially primarily affects the nail folds. The main non-dermatophyte moulds involved in onychomycosis are *Scopulariopsis* and *Scytalidium*, and such infections account for between 1.5 and 6% of nail infections. Many incidental non-dermatophytes and to a lesser extent yeasts may be isolated from non-sterile nail samples; these may become secondary colonisers.

In such countries as Australia, the UK and the USA, the incidence of onychomycosis has been estimated to be about 3% of the population, increasing to 5% in the elderly; some subgroups (such as miners, service personnel and sportspersons) have an incidence of up to 20% due to the use of communal showers and changing rooms. It is important to stress that fewer than 50% of dystrophic nails are of fungal aetiology and that it is therefore essential to establish a correct laboratory diagnosis by microscopy and/or culture before treating a patient with a systemic antifungal agent.

Identification of common dermatophytes

The identification of dermatophytes (Table 1.2) is primarily based on the microscopic morphology of the fungus. A good slide preparation is required and in some strains sporulation stimulation may be required. Culture characteristics, such as surface texture, topography and pigmentation, are variable and are therefore the least reliable criteria for identification. Clinical information such as the site, appearance of the lesion, geographic location, travel history, animal contacts and race is also important, especially in identifying rare non-sporulating species such as *M. audouinii, T. concentricum, T. schoenleinii* and many others.

Epidermophyton group

Epidermophyton floccosum is an anthropophilic dermatophyte with a worldwide distribution that often causes tinea pedis, tinea cruris and tinea corporis. Key

Table 1.2 Practical identification of common dermatophytes

Key features	Group	Common species
1) Smooth thin-walled macroconidia only, no microconidia; colonies a green-brown to khaki colour	Epidermophyton	E. floccosum
2) Macroconidia with rough walls present; microconidia may also be present	Microsporum	M. canis M. gypseum M. nanum
3) Microconidia present, smooth-walled macroconidia may or may not be present	Trichophyton	T. rubrum T. mentagrophytes T. tonsurans T. equinum
4) No conidia present, colonies sterile. Note: chlamydoconidia are non-diagnostic. Can you stimulate sporulation?	Non-sporulating Microsporum and Trichophyton species	M. audouinii M. ferrugineum T. verrucosum T. violaceum T. schoenleinii T. soudanense T. concentricum

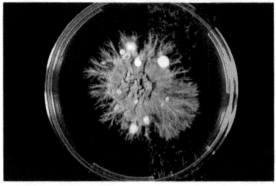

a

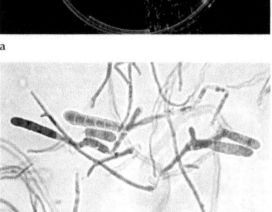

b

Figure 1.1
(a) Colonies of E. floccosum *are usually slow growing, greenish-brown or khaki in colour and have a suede-like surface, often raised and folded in the centre.*
(b) Macroconidia E. floccosum *are smooth, thin walled and club shaped, and often undergo rapid transformation into large chlamydoconidia. No microconidia are formed.*

features include characteristic greenish-brown or khaki-coloured cultures, the production of smooth, thin-walled, club-shaped macroconidia and the absence of microconidia (Figure 1.1(a) and (b)).

Microsporum group

In this group it is essential to observe macroconidia to make the identification. Difficulties may occur with non-sporulating strains of *M. canis* and with the differentiation between *M. canis* and *M. audouinii*.

Microsporum canis is a zoophilic dermatophyte of worldwide distribution that is a frequent cause of ringworm in humans, especially children. It invades hair, skin and, rarely, nails. Cats and dogs are the main sources of infection. Invaded hairs show an ectothrix infection and fluoresce a bright greenish-yellow under Wood's ultraviolet light. Key features include distinctive spindle-shaped macroconidia, culture characteristics (Figure 1.2(a) and (b)), and

5

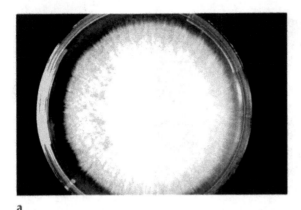

a

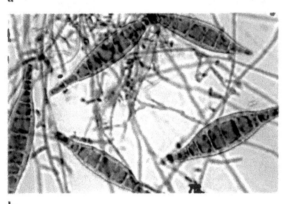

b

Figure 1.2
(a) Cultures of M. canis *are flat, spreading white to cream-coloured, with a dense cottony surface, and they usually have a bright golden-yellow to brownish-yellow reverse pigment.*
(b) Macroconidia of M. canis *are typically spindle shaped with 5–15 cells, verrucose, thick walled, and they often have a terminal knob.*

abundant growth and sporulation on polished rice grains and *in vitro* perforation of hair.

Microsporum gypseum is a geophilic fungus with a worldwide distribution that may cause infections in animals and humans, particularly children and rural workers during warm humid weather. It usually produces a single inflammatory skin or scalp lesion. Invaded hairs show an ectothrix infection but do not fluoresce under Wood's ultraviolet light. Key features include distinctive macroconidia and culture characteristics (Figure 1.3(a) and (b)).

Microsporum nanum is a zoophilic fungus frequently causing chronic non-inflammatory lesions in pigs and, rarely, causing tinea in humans; it is also present in the soil of pig-yards. Human infections are usually contracted directly from pigs or fomites. Invaded hairs typically show a sparse ectothrix or endothrix infection but do not fluoresce under Wood's ultraviolet light. The geographical distribution is worldwide. Key features include distinctive macroconidia and culture characteristics (Figure 1.4(a) and (b)).

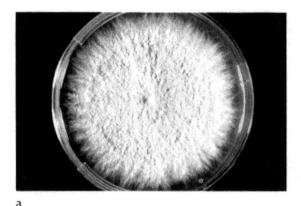

a

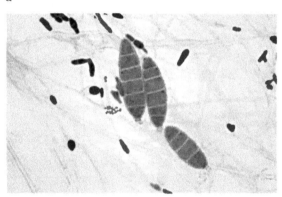

b

Figure 1.3
(a) Cultures of M. gypseum *are usually flat, suede-like to granular, with a deep cream to tawny-buff to pale cinnamon-coloured surface and a yellow-brown reverse pigment. (b) Macroconidia of* M. gypseum *are ellipsoidal, thin walled, verrucose and 4–6-celled.*

Microsporum cookei is a geophilic fungus that has been isolated from the hair of small mammals showing no clinical lesions. Infection has been reported in rodents, dogs and rarely in humans. It is not known to invade hair *in vivo*. It has a worldwide distribution.

Trichophyton group

In this group macroconidia are less distinctive and are often absent. Microconidia are more important and their shape, size and arrangement should be noted. Culture characteristics are also useful. Common species include *T. rubrum*, *T. mentagrophytes* and varieties, *T. tonsurans* and *T. equinum*. *Trichophyton verrucosum* may occasionally produce conidia on some media.

Trichophyton rubrum is an anthropophilic fungus that has become the most widely distributed dermatophyte of humans (Figure 1.5(a) and (b)). It

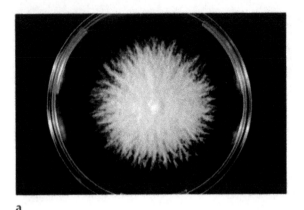

a

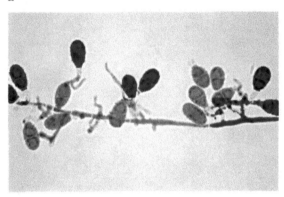

b

Figure 1.4
(a) Colonies of M. nanum *are flat, cream to buff in colour, with a suede-like to powdery surface texture and a dark reddish-brown reverse. (b) Macroconidia of* M. nanum *are small, ovoid to pyriform, mostly 2-celled with relatively thin, finely echinulate (rough) walls, and broad truncate bases.*

frequently causes chronic infections of skin, nails and, rarely, scalp. Granulomatous lesions may sometimes occur. Key features include culture characteristics, microscopic morphology and failure to perforate hair *in vitro.*

Trichophyton rubrum (granular strain) is a frequent cause of tinea corporis in southeast Asia and in Aborigines living in the Northern Territory of Australia. However, since the Vietnam War, it has been spread throughout the world, especially to those countries with returning troops or to those receiving refugees, where it has often been described as a new species. The granular strain of *T. rubrum* represents the parent strain of *T. rubrum* (downy type); the latter evolved by establishing a niche in feet (tinea pedis) when the former was imported into Europe at around the turn of the century. It should be stressed that intermediate strains between the two types do occur and that many culture and morphological characteristics overlap. Invaded hairs show ectothrix or endothrix infection but do not fluoresce under Wood's ultraviolet

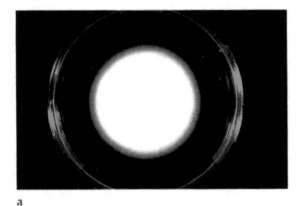

a

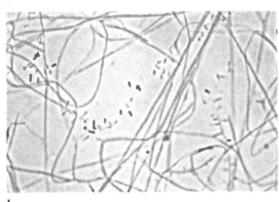

b

Figure 1.5
(a) Cultures of T. rubrum *are usually flat to slightly raised, white to cream, suede-like to downy, with a yellow-brown to wine-red reverse. (b) The microscopic morphology of* T. rubrum *showing the production of scanty to moderate numbers of slender clavate to pyriform microconidia. Macroconidia are usually absent.*

light. Key features include the presence of cigar-shaped macroconidia often with terminal appendages (Figure 1.6(a) and (b)).

Trichophyton mentagrophytes var. *interdigitale* is an anthropophilic fungus of worldwide distribution that is a common cause of tinea pedis (particularly the vesicular type), tinea corporis and sometimes superficial nail-plate invasion. It is not known to invade hair *in vivo*. Key features include culture characteristics, microscopic morphology and *in vitro* perforation of human hair. *Trichophyton mentagrophytes* var. *interdigitale* can be distinguished from *T. rubrum* and from other varieties of *T. mentagrophytes* by its culture characteristics and microscopic morphology on Sabouraud's dextrose agar and/or Lactritmel agar, and by its growth and colony morphology on Sabouraud's salt agar (Figure 1.7).

Trichophyton mentagrophytes var. *mentagrophytes* is the zoophilic form of *T. mentagrophytes* with a worldwide distribution and a wide range of animal hosts

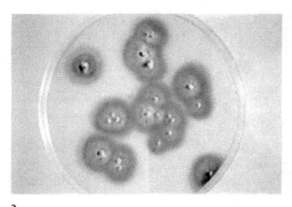

a

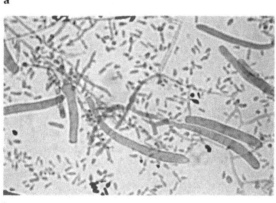

b

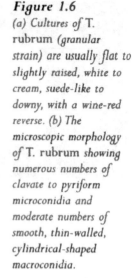

Figure 1.6
(a) Cultures of T. rubrum (granular strain) are usually flat to slightly raised, white to cream, suede-like to downy, with a wine-red reverse. (b) The microscopic morphology of T. rubrum showing numerous numbers of clavate to pyriform microconidia and moderate numbers of smooth, thin-walled, cylindrical-shaped macroconidia.

including mice, guinea-pigs, kangaroos, cats, horses, sheep and rabbits. It produces inflammatory skin or scalp lesions in humans, particularly in rural workers. Kerion of the scalp and beard may occur. Invaded hairs show an ectothrix infection but do not fluoresce under Wood's ultraviolet light. Key features include culture characteristics, microscopic morphology and clinical disease with known animal contacts (Figure 1.8(a) and (b)).

Other zoophilic varieties of *T. mentagrophytes* include *T. mentagrophytes* var. *quinckeanum* (mouse favus) and *T. mentagrophytes* var. *erinacei* (hedgehogs and epidermal mites).

Trichophyton tonsurans is an anthropophilic fungus with a worldwide distribution that causes inflammatory or chronic non-inflammatory finely scaling lesions of skin, nails and scalp. Invaded hairs show an endothrix infection and do not fluoresce under Wood's ultraviolet light. Key features include microscopic morphology, culture characteristics, endothrix invasion of hairs and partial thiamine requirement (Figure 1.9(a) and (b)).

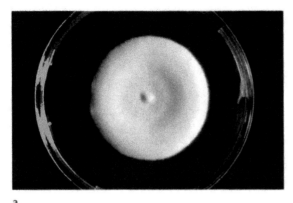

a

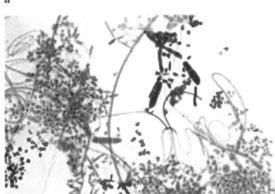

b

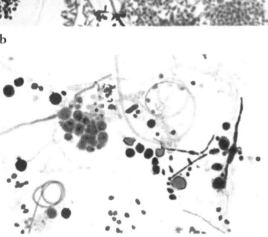

c

Figure 1.7
(a) Cultures of T. mentagrophytes *var.* interdigitale *are usually flat, white to cream in colour, with a powdery to suede-like surface and a yellowish to pinkish-brown reverse pigment, often becoming a darker red-brown with age.*
(b and c) The microscopic morphology of T. mentagrophytes *var.* interdigitale *showing numerous subspherical to pyriform microconidia, occasional spiral hyphae and spherical chlamydoconidia. There are occasional slender, clavate, smooth-walled macroconidia.*

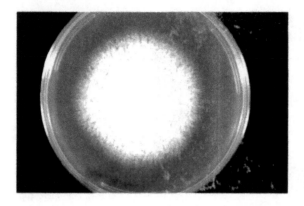

Figure 1.8
(a) Cultures of T. mentagrophytes var. mentagrophytes are generally flat, white to cream in colour, with a powdery to granular surface and a yellow-brown to reddish-brown reverse.

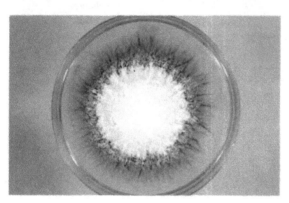

a

Trichophyton equinum is a zoophilic fungus causing ringworm in horses and rare infections in humans. It is of worldwide distribution except for var. autotrophicum, which is restricted to Australia and New Zealand. Invaded hairs show an ectothrix infection but do not fluoresce under Wood's ultraviolet light. Key features include microscopic morphology, culture characteristics, nicotinic acid requirement and clinical lesions in horses.

Non-sporulating Microsporum / Trichophyton species

Cultures of these species are usually sterile with no conidia present. Chlamydoconidia or other hyphal structures may be present but are non-diagnostic. In practice sporulation may need stimulation, e.g. to decide between non-sporing strains of *M. canis* or *T. rubrum*. Common species in this group include *M. audouinii*, *T. verrucosum* and *T. violaceum*. Less common ones are *T. concentricum*, *T. schoenleinii*, *T. soudanense* and *M. ferrugineum*.

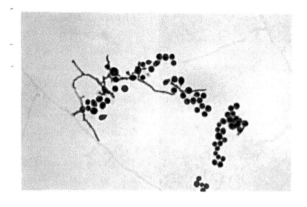

(b) The microscopic morphology of T. mentagrophytes *var.* mentagrophytes *showing numerous single-celled, spherical to subspherical microconidia, often in dense clusters. Varying numbers of spherical chlamydoconidia, spiral hyphae and smooth, thin-walled, clavate-shaped, multicelled macroconidia may also be present.*

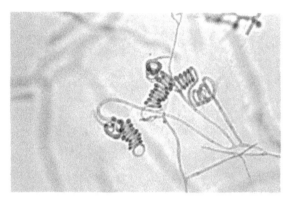

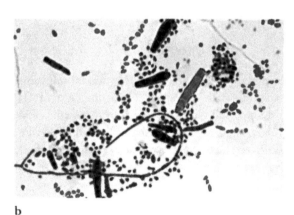

b

13

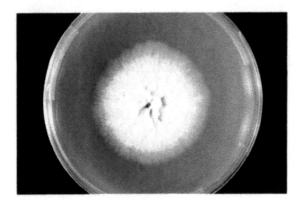

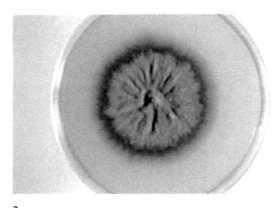

Figure 1.9
(a) Cultures of T. tonsurans *show considerable variation in texture and colour. They may be suede-like to powdery and flat with a raised centre or folded, often with radial grooves. The colour may vary from pale buff to yellow—the so-called sulfureum form which resembles* Epidermophyton floccosum—*to dark brown. The reverse colour varies from yellow-brown to reddish-brown to deep mahogany.*

a

Microsporum audouinii is an anthropophilic fungus causing non-inflammatory infections of the scalp and skin, especially in children. Once the cause of epidemics of tinea capitis in Europe and North America, this is now becoming less frequent. Invaded hairs show an ectothrix infection and usually fluoresce a bright greenish-yellow under Wood's ultraviolet light. Key features include the absence of conidia, poor or absence of growth on polished rice grains, inability to perforate hair *in vitro* and culture characteristics.

Trichophyton verrucosum is a zoophilic fungus causing ringworm in cattle (Figure 1.10(a) and (b)). Infections in humans result from direct contact with cattle or infected fomites and are usually highly inflammatory involving the scalp, beard or exposed, mainly hairy, areas of the body. Invaded hairs show an ectothrix infection, and fluorescence under Wood's ultraviolet light has been noted in cattle but not in humans. Geographic distribution is worldwide. Key features include culture characteristics and requirements for thiamine and inositol, large ectothrix invasion of hair, clinical lesions and history.

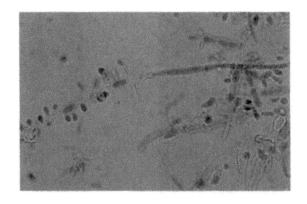

(b) The microscopic morphology of T. tonsurans *showing relatively broad, irregular, much branched hyphae with numerous septa. Numerous characteristic microconidia (varying in size and shape from long clavate to broad pyriform) are borne at right angles to the hyphae, which often remain unstained by lactophenol cotton blue. Very occasional smooth, thin-walled, irregular, clavate macroconidia may be present on some cultures. Numerous swollen giant forms of microconidia and chlamydoconidia are produced in older cultures.*

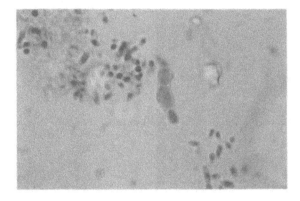

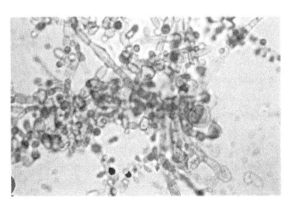

b

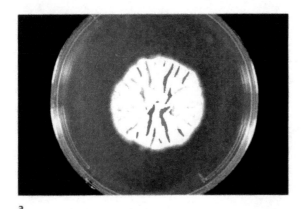

a

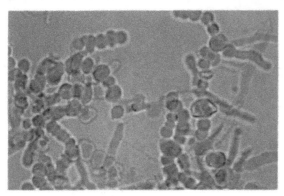

b

Figure 1.10
(a) Cultures of T. verrucosum *are slow growing, white to cream coloured, with a suede-like to velvety surface, a raised centre and a flat periphery with some submerged growth. Reverse pigment may vary from non-pigmented to yellow. (b) The microscopic morphology of* T. verrucosum *showing typical chains of chlamydoconidia when grown in brain heart infusion broth at 37°C.*

Trichophyton violaceum is an anthropophilic fungus causing inflammatory or chronic non-inflammatory finely scaling lesions of skin, nails, beard and scalp, producing the so-called 'black dot' tinea capitis. Distribution is worldwide, particularly in the Near East, eastern Europe, the former USSR and north Africa. Key features include culture characteristics, endothrix hair invasion and a partial requirement for thiamine, which separates this organism from *T. gourvillii*, *T. rubrum* and other species that may produce purple-pigmented colonies.

Trichophyton schoenleinii is an anthropophilic fungus causing favus in humans. Favus is a chronic, scarring form of tinea capitis characterised by saucer-shaped crusted lesions or scutula and permanent hair loss. Invaded hairs remain intact and fluoresce a pale greenish-yellow under Wood's ultraviolet light. Favus is common in Eurasia and Africa. Key features include clinical history, culture characteristics and microscopic morphology showing favic chandeliers (Figure 1.11(a) and (b)).

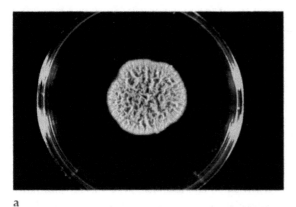

a

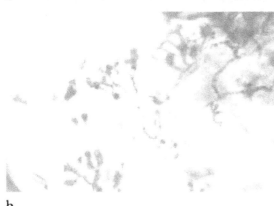

b

Figure 1.11
(a) Cultures of T. schoenleinii *are slow growing, waxy or suede-like, with a deeply folded honey-comb-like thallus and some subsurface growth. The thallus is cream coloured to yellow to orange-brown. Cultures are difficult to maintain in their typical convoluted form, and rapidly become flat and downy. (b) The microscopic morphology of* T. schoenleinii *showing characteristic antler 'nail head' hyphae also known as 'favic chandeliers'.*

Trichophyton soudanense is an anthropophilic fungus that is a frequent cause of tinea capitis in Africa. Invaded hairs show an endothrix infection but do not fluoresce under Wood's ultraviolet light. Distribution is mainly in Africa with occasional isolates in Europe, Brazil and the USA. Key features include clinical history, culture characteristics and microscopic morphology showing reflexive hyphal branching and endothrix invasion of hair.

Trichophyton concentricum is an anthropophilic fungus that causes chronic widespread non-inflammatory tinea corporis known as tinea imbricata because of the concentric rings of scaling it produces. It is not known to invade hair. Infections among Europeans are rare. Distribution is restricted to the Pacific Islands of Oceania, southeast Asia and Central and South America. Key features include the clinical signs, geographical distribution and culture characteristics.

Microsporum ferrugineum is an anthropophilic fungus causing epidemic juvenile tinea capitis in humans. The clinical features are similar to those of infections caused by *M. audouinii*. Invaded hairs show an ectothrix infection and fluoresce a greenish-yellow under Wood's ultraviolet light. It is reported from Asia (including China and Japan), the former USSR, eastern Europe and Africa. Key mycological features include clinical history, culture characteristics and distinctive 'bamboo' hyphae.

Identification of yeast-like fungi

The identification of yeast-like fungi is primarily based on physiological and biochemical tests, including fermentation and assimilation of various substrates based on those used at the Centraalbureau voor Schimmelcultures, Delft, The Netherlands (Kreger-Van Rij, *The yeasts: a taxonomic study*, Elsevier Science Publishers: Amsterdam, 1984). Reliable commercially available yeast identification kits are the API 20C AUX, ATB 32C, MicroScan and Vitek systems. The germ tube test is also useful for the rapid identification of *Candida albicans*, and morphological studies (Dalmau plate culture) are also helpful.

Candida

Several species of *Candida* may be aetiological agents in humans, most commonly *Candida albicans* and, rarely, *C. tropicalis*, *C. krusei*, *C. parapsilosis*, *C. guilliermondii*, *C. kefyr* (*C. pseudotropicalis*) and *C. (Torulopsis) glabrata*. All are ubiquitous and occur naturally on humans, especially *C. albicans*, which is recognised as a commensal of the mouth, gastrointestinal tract and vagina.

The genus *Candida* is characterised by globose to elongate yeast-like cells or blastoconidia that reproduce by multilateral budding. Most *Candida* species are also characterised by the presence of well developed pseudohyphae. However, this characteristic may be absent, especially in those species formally included in the genus *Torulopsis*.

Candida albicans (Figure 1.12(a) and (b)) occurs naturally as a commensal of mucous membranes and in the digestive tract of humans and animals. It accounts for up to 70% of *Candida* species isolated from sites of infection and has been reported as a causative agent of all types of candidiasis. Environmental isolations are usually from sources contaminated by human or animal excreta, such as polluted water, soil, air and plants.

Candida dublinensis has recently been recognised from the oral cavity of HIV infected patients and is most frequently implicated in cases of recurrent infection following antifungal drug treatment. Phenotypically, isolates are very similar to *C. albicans* in that isolates produce both germ tubes and chlamydoconidia. However, they have unusual carbohydrate assimilation patterns and grow poorly or not at all at 42 °C.

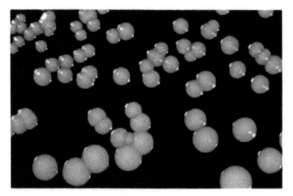

Figure 1.12
(a) A culture of C. albicans *on Sabouraud's dextrose agar showing typical cream-coloured, smooth-surfaced waxy colonies. (b) The microscopic morphology of* C. albicans *showing budding spherical to ovoid blastoconidia.*

a

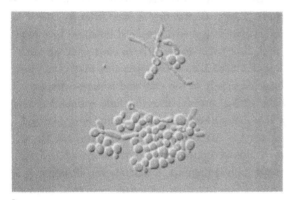

b

Candida (Torulopsis) glabrata is one of the most common yeast species to be found on the body surface and is often isolated as an incidental finding from skin and urine. It has been implicated as an 'opportunistic' cause of both superficial and systemic infections, especially in immunocompromised patients, and it has been isolated from patients with septicaemia, pyelonephritis, pulmonary infections, endocarditis and hyperalimentation. The incidence of *Candida glabrata* has doubled over the last 5 years and it now accounts for 8–10% of yeast infections.

Candida guilliermondii has been isolated from numerous human infections, mostly of cutaneous origin. Systemic infections are rare, although they have been reported in patients with aplastic anaemia. *C. guilliermondii* has also been isolated from normal skin and from sea water, faeces of animals, fig wasps, buttermilk, leather, fish and beer.

Candida kefyr (= *Candida pseudotropicalis*) is a rare cause of candidiasis and is usually associated with superficial cutaneous manifestations rather than systemic disease. It has been isolated from nails and lung infections. Environmental isolations have been made from cheese and dairy products.

Candida krusei is regularly associated with some forms of infant diarrhoea and occasionally with systemic disease. It has also been reported to colonise the gastrointestinal, respiratory and urinary tracts of patients with granulocytopenia. Environmental isolations have been made from beer, milk products, skin, faeces of animals and birds and pickle brine.

Candida lusitaniae has been isolated from several cases of disseminate candidiasis, including septicaemia and pyelonephritis. It has also been reported to colonise the human respiratory, gastrointestinal and urinary tracts and many strains have proven to be resistant to amphotericin B. *C. lusitaniae* was first isolated from the alimentary tract of warm-blooded animals and environmental isolations have been made from cornmeal, citrus peel, fruit juices and milk from cows with mastitis.

Candida parapsilosis is an opportunistic human pathogen that may cause both superficial cutaneous infections (especially of the nail) and systemic disease (especially endocarditis). Other clinical manifestations include endophthalmitis and fungaemia. Environmental isolations have been made from intertidal and oceanic waters, pickle brine, cured meats, olives and normal skin, and faeces.

Candida tropicalis is a major cause of septicaemia and disseminated candidiasis, especially in patients with lymphoma, leukaemia and diabetes. It is the second most frequently encountered medical pathogen, next to *C. albicans*, and is also found as part of the normal human mucocutaneous flora. Environmental isolations have been made from faeces, shrimp, kefir and soil.

Malassezia furfur (Pityrosporum)

M. furfur is the causative agent of pityriasis versicolor and is also implicated as a causative agent of seborrhoeic dermatitis and dandruff. It has also been recovered in blood cultures from neonate and adult patients undergoing lipid replacement therapy. Diagnosis requires special culture media, and blood drawn back through the catheter is the preferred specimen. Culture of the catheter tip is also recommended. *M. furfur* is characterised by globose, oblong-ellipsoidal to cylindrical yeast cells (Figure 1.13(a) and (b)). Reproduction is by budding on a broad base and from the same site at one pole (unipolar). It is a lipophilic yeast; therefore *in vitro* growth must be stimulated by natural oils or other fatty substances.

Identification of non–dermatophyte moulds

The identification of non-dermatophyte moulds is primarily based on microscopic morphology. Culture characteristics, although less reliable, may

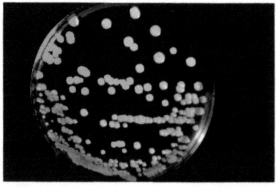

a

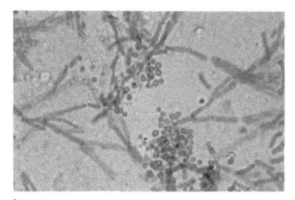

b

Figure 1.13
(a) Colonies of Malassezia furfur *on Dixon's agar. (b) Skin scrapings taken from patients with pityriasis versicolor stain rapidly when mounted in 10% KOH, glycerol and Parker ink solution, and show characteristic clusters of thick-walled, round, budding yeast-like cells and short angular hyphal forms up to 8 μm in diameter (average diameter 4 μm). These microscopic features are diagnostic for the causative agent* Malassezia furfur, *and culture preparations are usually not necessary.*

also be useful. These include surface texture, topography and pigmentation, reverse pigmentation and growth at 37 °C. Non-dermatophyte moulds reported as causative agents of skin infection and/or onychomycosis include the following:

Acremonium   A rare cause of onychomycosis, mycetoma, arthritis, osteomyelitis, peritonitis, endocarditis and pneumonia. Species include *A. falciforme, A. kiliense, A. recifei, A. alabamensis, A. roseo-griseum* and *A. strictum.* They are found mostly in plant debris and soil.

Aspergillus   Several species of *Aspergillus* have been reported as opportunistic human pathogens, notably *A. fumigatus, A. flavus, A. niger, A. nidulans* and *A. terreus.* They are cosmopolitan moulds from soil and plant debris, but they will grow on a wide variety of substrates.

Chrysosporium   Species of *Chrysosporium* are occasionally isolated from skin and nail scrapings, especially from feet, but because they are common soil

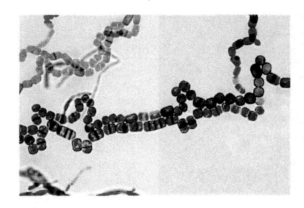

Figure 1.14
Scytalidium *anamorph of* Nattrassia mangiferae *showing chains of 1–2-celled, darkly pigmented arthroconidia.*

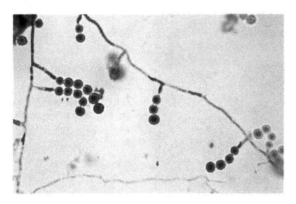

Figure 1.15
Scopulariopsis brevicaulis *showing chains of single-celled conidia produced by a specialised condiogenous cell called an annellide.*

saprophytes they are usually considered as contaminants. There are about 22 species of *Chrysosporium*. Several are keratinophilic with some also being thermotolerant. Cultures may closely resemble some dermatophytes, especially *Trichophyton mentagrophytes*.

Fusarium Several species of *Fusarium* have been reported as opportunistic pathogens of humans causing cutaneous and subcutaneous infections, mycotic keratitis, endophthalmitis, osteomyelitis and arthritis following traumatic implantation. *F. oxysporum, F. solani* and *F. moniliforme* are common soil fungi with a worldwide distribution.

Geotrichum candidum A rare opportunistic pathogen causing bronchial and pulmonary infections; oral, vaginal, cutaneous and gastrointestinal infections are also reported. This is a common fungus with a worldwide distribution.

Nattrassia mangiferae (synonym *Hendersonula toruloidea*) This is a rare agent of onychomycosis and superficial skin infections, especially in tropical regions (Figure 1.14).

Phaeoannellomyces werneckii   This is a causative agent of tinea nigra and a common saprophytic fungus from soil, compost and wood in humid tropical regions.

Scopulariopsis   Most members of this genus are soil fungi. However, *S. brevicaulis* has been reported as a causative agent of onychomycosis and of hyalohyphomycosis in immunosuppressed patients (Figure 1.15).

Laboratory diagnosis of dermatophytosis

Specimen collection and transport

For a laboratory diagnosis, clinicians should be aware of the need to generate an adequate amount of suitable clinical material. Unfortunately many specimens submitted are either of an inadequate amount or are not appropriate for a definitive diagnosis. Remember, the laboratory requires enough tissue to perform both microscopy and culture.

Hairs for dermatophytosis and for white and black piedra

In patients with suspected ringworm of the scalp, the broken hair stumps near the advancing border of the lesions should be epilated with a pair of forceps or flat-edged tweezers. The hairs and scale should be removed so that the hair roots can be seen extending beyond the edge of the forceps. Infected hair roots appear as a solid white colour whereas normal hairs are more transparent.

Hairs with an endothrix type of invasion are usually so packed with spores and digested by the fungus that they become twisted and fractured when they reach the surface of the scalp. In these cases the forceps must be firmly pressed and scraped into any scale present, which is then removed in the hope it will contain broken fragments of infected hairs.

In kerion of the scalp or skin, specimens are often difficult to obtain as hairs may be spontaneously expelled due to the acute inflammation. Sometimes broken hairs can be epilated from the edge of the lesions, and a swab of pus should also be collected for both mycological and bacterial culture. Although many kerions are entirely the result of a fungus, secondary bacterial infection is common.

In patients with suspected piedra, collect hairs – preferably those with visible nodules along their shafts.

Skin scrapings for dermatophytosis, candidiasis, pityriasis versicolor and tinea nigra

In patients with suspected dermatophytosis of the skin (tinea or ringworm), any ointments or other local applications present should first be removed with an Alcowipe. Using a blunt scalpel, tweezers or a curette, firmly scrape the lesion, particularly at the advancing border. A curette is safe and useful for collecting specimens from babies, young children and awkward sites, such as interdigital spaces. If multiple lesions are present choose the most recent for scrapings, as old loose scale is often unsatisfactory. Any small vellus hairs when present within the lesions should be epilated. The roof of any fresh vesicles should be removed as the fungus is often plentiful in this site, especially in cases of vesicular tinea pedis.

In patients with suspected candidiasis, the young 'satellite' lesions that have not undergone exfoliation are more likely to yield positive results if they are present. Otherwise the advancing scaly border should be scraped. When lesions in the flexures are moist and very inflamed, it is more satisfactory and less painful to roll a moistened swab firmly over the surface.

In patients with suspected pityriasis versicolor, Sellotape strippings may also be taken by firmly applying a piece of the tape across the lesion and then quickly removing it. Skin scrapings as for tinea should also be performed.

In patients with suspected tinea nigra, scrape the lesions with a curette or blunt scalpel as for tinea.

Note: Do not overlook the use of swabs in mycological investigations. Following the collection of skin scales, all scraped lesions should be firmly rubbed with a swab moistened in either BHI or Sabouraud's broth.

Nail scrapings for dermatophytosis and candidiasis

In patients with suspected dermatophytosis of the nails (onychomycosis), the nail plate should be pared and scraped using a blunt scalpel until the crumbling white degenerating portion is reached. Any white keratin debris beneath the free edge of the nail (hyponychium) should also be collected. Chronic paronychia is often invaded by *Candida* infection and in these cases a swab moistened in sterile saline should be firmly rolled several times around the nail fold; the liquid is forced beneath the fold and is then sucked back on to the swab.

Special notes for onychomycosis

As the treatment of dermatophyte onychomycosis generally requires long-term therapy with an oral antifungal, it is essential to diagnose the infection accurately.

An inaccurate negative diagnosis will lead to continual disfigurement and discomfort for the patient, whereas an inaccurate positive diagnosis may lead to a long-term, useless and expensive treatment regime. Clinicians and laboratory staff alike often have a misconception that the diagnosis of onychomycosis is simple; in theory it should be – but in practice it is often difficult!

A recent survey of 83 laboratories in Australia reported an average positive strike rate of 45% for nail samples examined by both direct microscopy and culture. A total of 32 000 nail samples were processed with 14 200 reported as positive; 10–40% were positive by microscopy alone and 10–30% were positive by culture alone. The high laboratory error rate is most often due to sampling errors associated with an inadequate specimen and/or in splitting the sample to perform both microscopy and culture. A positive microscopy result showing fungal hyphae and/or arthroconidia is generally sufficient for the diagnosis of dermatophytosis but gives no indication as to the species of fungus involved. A negative culture result may also be due to the presence of non-viable hyphal elements in the distal region of the nail. Therefore, it is essential to perform both direct microscopy and culture on all specimens, and repeat collections should always be considered in cases of suspected dermatophytosis with negative laboratory reports. When laboratories were asked about the quality of the specimens they received, 10–30% were described as inadequate, 50–60% as adequate, while only 10–20% were described as excellent. Another interesting fact to emerge from this survey was that the better performing laboratories spent between 20 and 30 minutes setting up and examining each specimen. Laboratory managers also need to recognise that the current diagnostic methods are labour intensive and require special interpretative skills, especially when examining direct microscopic slides of clinical material and in the identification of fungal cultures.

Mailing of skin, scalp and nail specimens to the laboratory

Skin and nail specimens may be scraped directly on to special black cards (or X-ray black paper), which makes it easier to see how much material has been collected. This method also provides the ideal conditions for transporting the specimens to the laboratory (Figure 1.16 (a) and (b)). These black collection cards may be sealed and mailed directly to the laboratory for processing. Fungal elements in skin, hair and nail specimens will remain viable for weeks in these cards. The greater the amount of specimen, the greater the chance of obtaining a positive result from both direct microscopy and culture! A variety of collection tools has been used in attempts to gain better specimens, and these include dental/engraving drills, household drills, punch biopsy instruments, bone or skin ring curettes and blunt scalpel blades.

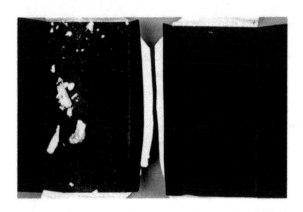

Figure 1.16
Nail specimens on black transport cards. (Left) An adequate collection. (Right) A grossly inadequate specimen.

Direct microscopy

Direct microscopic examination of skin, hair or nail scrapings provides vital information. Often a presumptive diagnosis is possible with microscopy, which is of particular importance if laboratory proof is required before treatment may commence. A wet mount is usually made using either (1) 10% potassium hydroxide (KOH) with Parker ink; (2) 10% KOH–dimethylsulphoxide (DMSO); or (3) calcofluor white. Nail specimens may need to be shaved into smaller pieces using a scalpel blade prior to examination.

Potassium hydroxide (KOH) with Parker ink

This is the most widely used technique but it may take time for the specimen to clear and stain. However, preparations last a long time and may be kept until the culture result is known. Dissolve the 10 gm of potassium hydroxide (KOH) in 80 ml of distilled water, then add 10 ml of glycerol and 10 ml of Parker Quink permanent blue ink. The glycerol prevents crystallisation of the reagent and prevents the specimen from drying out. Mount a small portion of the specimen in a drop of stain, cover with a coverslip, squash the preparation with the butt of the inoculation needle and then blot off the excess fluid. Gently heat by passing through a flame two or three times. Do not boil. When the specimen has cleared, which may take up to 20 minutes for skin scrapings to several hours for nail scrapings, examine microscopically for the presence of faintly blue-stained fungal elements.

Note: Negative specimens should be kept and re-examined the next day to avoid reporting false-negative results because of the delayed clearance and staining of the specimen.

Potassium hydroxide–dimethylsulphoxide (KOH–DMSO) preparation

This method gives a more rapid maceration and clearing than potassium hydroxide alone. However, preparations do not keep. Using a safety pipette, add 40 ml of dimethylsulphoxide (DMSO) to 60 ml of distilled water and then dissolve 10 gm of KOH into the solution. Mount a small portion of the specimen as described above but do *not* heat the preparation. The mount must be examined within 20 minutes. Using low light, examine microscopically for the presence of unstained refractile fungal elements.

Calcofluor white with 10% potassium hydroxide (KOH)

This is a very rapid and sensitive method. However, a fluorescence microscope fitted with filters to give an excitation with ultraviolet light below 400 nm wavelength is required. Calcofluor white (M2R powder from Polysciences) or Blankophor BA (from Bayer) are used as whitening agents by the paper industry and selectively bind to cellulose and chitin. The dye fluoresces as it is exposed to ultraviolet light. Prepare two solutions: (1) dissolve 10 gm of KOH in 90 ml distilled water and then add 10 ml of glycerol; (2) dissolve 0.1 gm of calcofluor white powder in 100 ml of distilled water by gentle heating. Mix one drop of each solution on the centre of a clean microscope slide and mount a small portion of the specimen as described above. Gently heat the slide and examine microscopically for the presence of fungal elements that fluoresce a chalk-white or brilliant apple-green colour, depending on the filters used.

Interpretation of direct microscopy results

The recognition of fungal elements in skin and nail specimens is a technique that requires considerable experience and expertise. Fungal elements within the specimen may be scanty in number and thus be missed by the inexperienced, resulting in false-negatives.

It is important to be able to recognise the difference between ectothrix and endothrix hair infection as all endothrix infections are caused by anthropophilic dermatophytes, whereas ectothrix infections are mostly zoophilic in nature (Figures 1.17 and 1.18).

In skin scrapings the presence of thick-walled, broad-based, budding yeast-like cells and short pseudohyphae ('spaghetti and meatballs') is diagnostic for *Malassezia (Pityrosporum) furfur* (Figure 1.13b). In skin and nail specimens, the presence of hyaline, septate fungal hyphae (often forming arthroconidia)

27

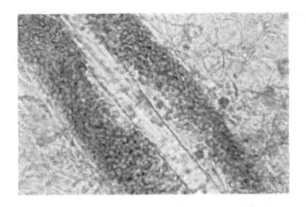

Figure 1.17
Ectothrix hair invasion showing the formation of arthroconidia on the outside of the hair shaft. The cuticle of the hair is destroyed.

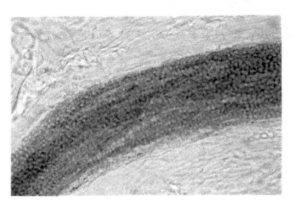

Figure 1.18
Endothrix hair invasion showing the development of arthroconidia within the hair shaft only. The cuticle of the hair remains intact.

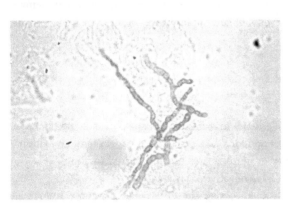

Figure 1.19
Skin scraping showing hyaline, septate hyphae diagnostic for a dermatophyte.

should be considered significant and is presumptive of a dermatophyte infection (Figure 1.19). In skin and nail specimens, the presence of budding yeast cells and pseudohyphae is also significant and is presumptive of a *Candida* infection (Figure 1.20).

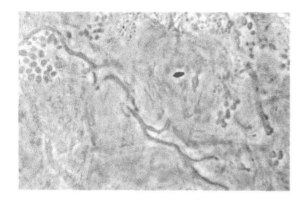

Figure 1.20
Skin scraping from superficial candidiasis showing clusters of budding yeast cells and branching pseudohyphae.

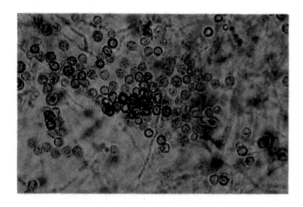

Figure 1.21
Nail scrapings showing clusters of conidia typical of Scopulariopsis brevicaulis.

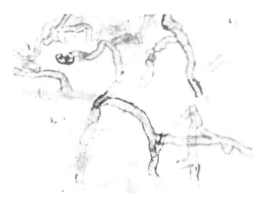

Figure 1.22
Nail scrapings showing the presence of thick-walled, dematiaceous, brown-pigmented septate hyphae typical of Nattrassia mangiferae (Hendersonula toruloidea).

In nails infected by *Scopulariopsis*, characteristic conidia are usually seen within the nail body (Figure 1.21). Similarly with *Nattrassia mangiferae* (*Hendersonula toruloidea*), the presence of thick-walled, dematiaceous, brown-pigmented septate hyphae can be detected by direct microscopy (Figure 1.22).

29

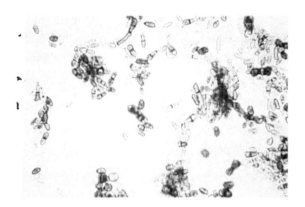

Figure 1.23
Skin scrapings mounted
in 10% KOH showing
pigmented brown to dark
olivaceous (dematiaceous)
septate hyphal elements
and 2-celled yeast cells
producing annelloconidia
typical of
Phaeoannellomyces
(Exophiala) werneckii.

In skin scrapings from patients with suspected tinea nigra, the presence of dark olivaceous septate hyphal elements and 2-celled yeast cells producing annelloconidia is significant (Figure 1.23).

Culture

For culture, specimens are usually inoculated on to Sabouraud's dextrose agar containing cycloheximide (actidione), chloramphenicol, gentamicin and yeast extract. Other suitable media include dermasel agar (Oxoid), mycobiotic agar (Difco) and dermatophyte test medium. However, non-dermatophyte moulds and yeasts will not grow in the presence of cycloheximide (actidione), and duplicate plates will need to be set up to isolate these fungi.

It is useful to cut the skin scales or small pieces of nail into the agar. Cultures may be incubated at 26–30 °C for 4 weeks and should be examined regularly. Fungal growths should be identified and significant isolates reported as soon as possible.

Interpretation of culture results

Significant culture results include the growth of a dermatophyte and the growth of any mould or yeast associated with a matching direct microscopy. Interpretation of culture results in onychomycosis is often more problematic. Most cases of onychomycosis occur in the toenails rather than the fingernails, and dermatophytes are the most important pathogens. *Trichophyton rubrum* is the most common causative agent, followed by *T. mentagrophytes* var. *interdigitale* and *Epidermophyton floccosum*. Data obtained from a recent study on

Table 1.3 Routine laboratory turnaround times

Organism	Direct microscopy	Culture	Identification	Total
C. albicans	24 hrs	48 hrs	3 hrs	2–3 days
Other yeasts	24 hrs	48 hrs	72–96 hrs	5–8 days
Dermatophytes	24 hrs	14–28 days	1–28 days	14–42 days
Other moulds	24 hrs	5–28 days	1–28 days	5–42 days

118 patients with onychomycosis showed that 81% were infected with *Trichophyton rubrum*, 16% with *T. mentagrophytes* var. *interdigitale*, 2% with *T. tonsurans* and 1% with *Epidermophyton floccosum*. However, dystrophic nails harbour a large flora of saprophytic fungi, yeasts and bacteria associated with a non-sterile site. Therefore the isolation of a yeast or other mould without supporting microscopy is not significant. Contaminant fungi may be isolated from two-thirds of patients examined, but successive sampling of the same nail will rarely demonstrate the same contaminant.

The key elements for the diagnosis of onychomycosis are thus the collection of an adequate specimen and the correct processing and interpretation of both microscopy and culture results. Given the common occurrence of incidental contaminants from non-sterile nail samples, it would be useful for clinicians if laboratory reports included a comment on the likely significance of a culture result, as well as the result itself. Repeat collections may also be necessary to detect the presence of a dermatophyte in nail specimens as most contaminant fungi will overgrow or mask the presence of a dermatophyte in culture.

Routine turnaround times for direct microscopy should be less than 24 hours. However, culture may take several weeks (Table 1.3).

2 DERMATOMYCOSES

Tinea pedis

Tinea pedis (Figures 2.1–2.6) is a fungal infection of the foot that may involve the toe webs. It is often called athlete's foot and is the most common fungal infection. Hot, moist climates are particularly conducive to clinical manifestation. Genetic predisposition is known to occur for plantar type of tinea pedis.

Tinea pedis occurs in three principal forms.

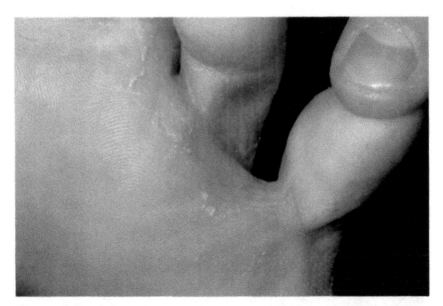

Figure 2.1
Tinea pedis—interdigital quiescent form. The objective findings are slight scaling only, as remnants of small vesicles. Itching may be troublesome even in minor forms of tinea pedis as here. The causative agent was T. rubrum.

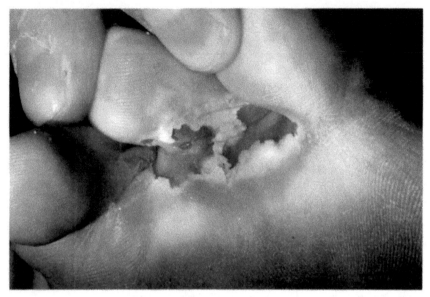

Figure 2.2

Tinea pedis. In the more severe form of interdigital tinea pedis, maceration and secondary bacterial infection may occur. As here, the causative fungus is T. rubrum. *Topical therapy with antibacterial baths and compresses may be necessary, followed by appropriate antifungal therapy.*

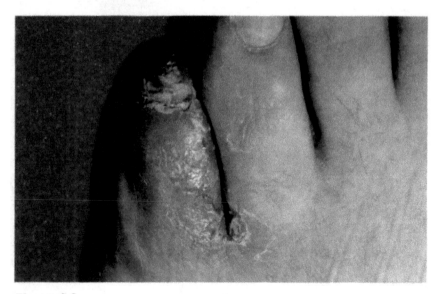

Figure 2.3

Tinea pedis from above: there is some secondary eczematous change. It can be seen as a sign of normal host immune response to an invading organism. In severely itching cases, a shorter course of topical corticosteroid cream may be combined with antifungal therapy.

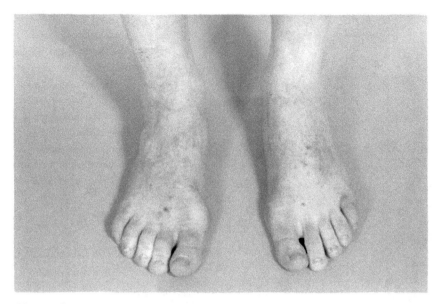

Figure 2.4
Tinea pedis—bilateral lesions on the dorsum of both feet.

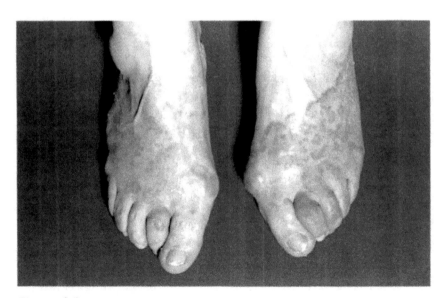

Figure 2.5
Tinea pedis—inflammatory type with active edge.

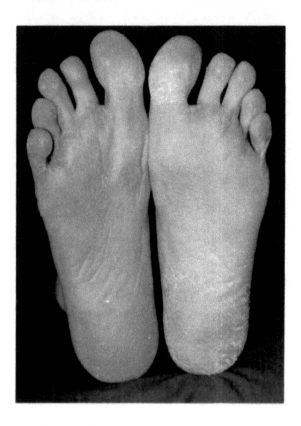

Figure 2.6
Tinea pedis—plantar type. Quite commonly the plantar mycosis caused by T. rubrum *is unilateral, as in this case of the left foot. Often this form of dermatophyte infection spreads to the nails. Topical therapy is usually not sufficient to eradicate plantar* T. rubrum *infection.*

'Mocassin' type

This infection is most commonly associated with *T. rubrum*, and is characterised by diffuse scaling, lack of inflammation and extreme chronicity. This may be the only manifestation of tinea pedis: the patient complains of dryness of the sole or soles, which are resistant to emollients. In its mildest form it may only manifest as small scaly 'rings' that are similar to healed vesicles. It often also affects only one foot.

Interdigital

Scaling, itching, maceration, sogginess and fissuring of the interdigital spaces are the characteristics of this form of tinea pedis. The fourth web space is most commonly involved but in severe cases all the interdigital spaces may be affected. Interdigital tinea pedis is the most common type of human fungal infection. Occasionally it spreads to the upper aspect of the foot, which presents with a reddish, scaly advancing border.

Secondary infections due to bacteria may further complicate the clinical picture. These may show as pain, lymphangitis or erysipelas.

Vesicular type

The common sites of infection are the instep, the sole, the heel and the ball of the foot. The vesicles may fuse to form blisters that contain yellowish, gelatinous fluid. Relapses are common, particularly if the condition is not treated for extended periods of time. This is particularly true of the mocassin form.

Some of the relatively common conditions that may mimic tinea pedis are shown in Figures 2.7–2.14.

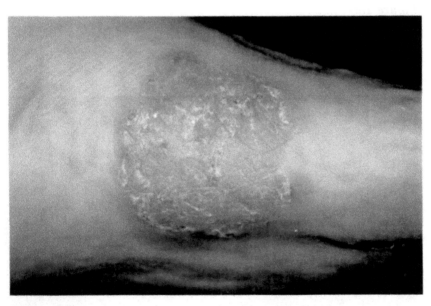

Figure 2.7
Tinea pedis—differential diagnosis: chronic eczema.

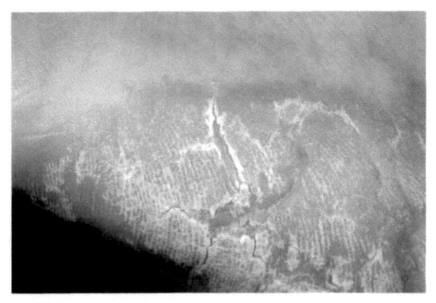

Figure 2.8
Tinea pedis—differential diagnosis: psoriasis in plantar-lateral aspect of the foot.

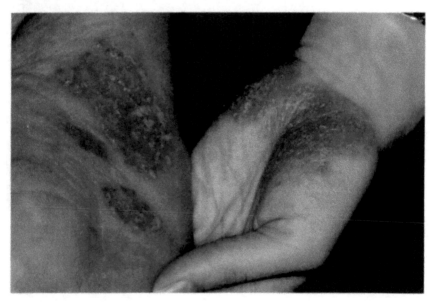

Figure 2.9
Tinea pedis—differential diagnosis: palmplantar pustulosis (PPP). This is a relatively common bilateral, chronic dermatosis of unknown aetiology with exceptional therapy resistance.

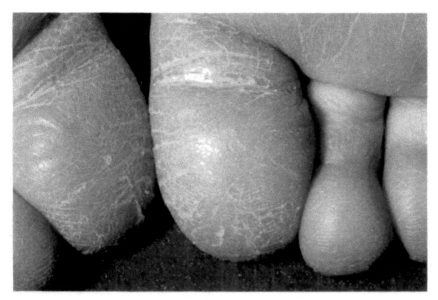

Figure 2.10

Tinea pedis—differential diagnosis: juvenile plantar dermatosis. Juvenile plantar dermatosis (commonly seen as a variation of atopic dermatitis) primarily affects the contact surface of the big toe and the front part of the plantar skin. The skin is dry, chapped and often painfully fissured. Similar changes are often found on the distal volar skin of the fingers.

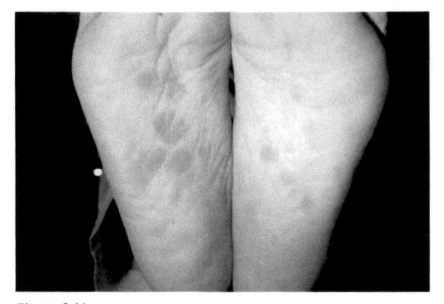

Figure 2.11

Tinea pedis—differential diagnosis: lues II (secondary syphilis). Macular lesions in plantar (and palmar) skin. Positive serology confirms the diagnosis.

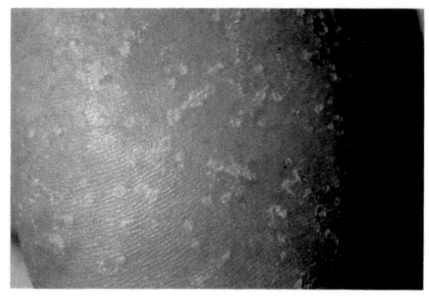

Figure 2.12

Tinea pedis—differential diagnosis: pitted keratolysis. Pitted keratolysis may be confused with the plantar type of tinea. The scales in plantar tinea are very superficial; there are no crypts of the pitted keratolysis type. Pitted keratolysis is caused by erythrasma bacteria and is one of the typical skin signs found in HIV infection.

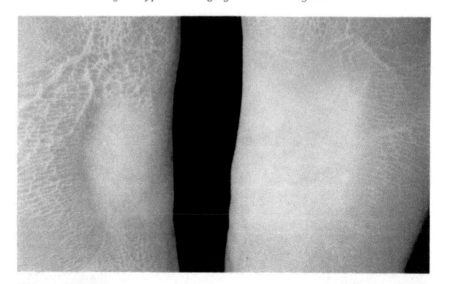

Figure 2.13

Tinea pedis—differential diagnosis: hereditary keratoderma (Thost–Unna). Hereditary palmo-plantar hyperkeratosis (Thost–Unna type) affects the hands and feet in symmetric fashion. The thick hyperkeratosis does not affect the central part of the plantar skin, and there is no sign of inflammatory reaction. Secondary invasion by fungi is possible.

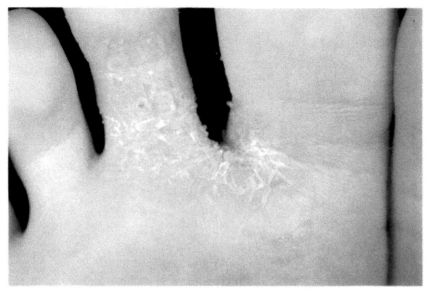

Figure 2.14

Tinea pedis—differential diagnosis: atopic dermatitis in the first and second toe webs. Fungal infection in the feet most commonly affects the lateral toe clefts. This patient has atopic dermatitis in addition to the most typical locations; it is also present in the first toe cleft. The typical lesions of atopic dermatitis in other skin areas and negative mycology confirm the diagnosis.

Tinea cruris

Tinea cruris (Figures 2.15–2.18) is intertriginous, involving the groin, perineum or perianal regions. Tinea cruris is found in all areas of the world but is more common in humid tropical conditions. It occurs more frequently in men than women.

With topical or systemic therapy, prognosis is good. Maintaining dryness with regular absorbent powders might help to prevent relapses. Several conditions that may mimic tinea cruris are shown in Figures 2.19–2.22.

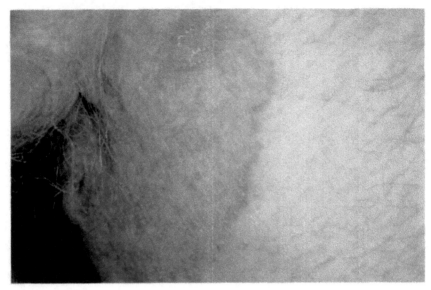

Figure 2.15

Tinea cruris—normal. Typical fungal infection in the inguinal region. The active border is scaly, raised and red. In this case there is secondary spread from a hair follicle. The follicular infection may form fungal pustules. The causative agent was proved to be T. rubrum.

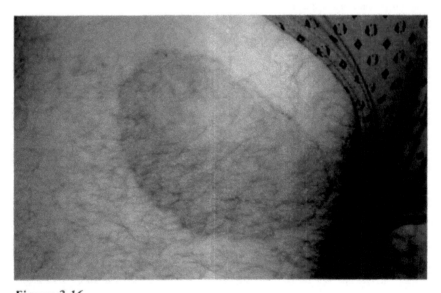

Figure 2.16

Tinea cruris—outside the inguinal fold. Fungal infection in the groin is usually centred in the inguinal fold, but may appear on the skin of the leg as in this case. The even redness without marked accentuation at the transition to normal skin is also different from the usual manifestation of this infection. The causative agent is T. rubrum.

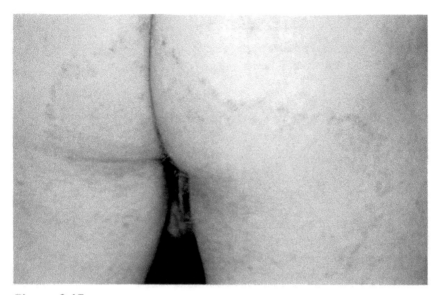

Figure 2.17

Tinea cruris—spreading to the gluteal region. Occasionally the not-unusual male-type of tinea in the inguinal region spreads more widely, and also into the gluteal region. The reddish central area with a more accentuated, slowly spreading, scaly margin is a typical feature. Positive mycology confirms the diagnosis. The simultaneous infection of the toe webs or/and plantar surfaces is common.

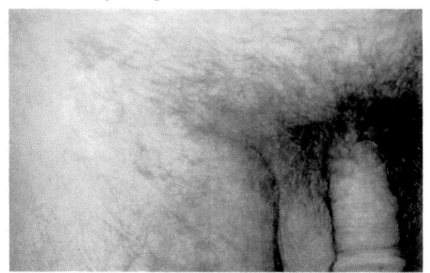

Figure 2.18

Tinea cruris—tinea incognito (steroid-induced changes). Tinea incognito is the result of the inappropriate use of topical corticosteroids in fungal infection. The typical features of ringworms are partially hidden, which can often further delay the correct fungal diagnosis.

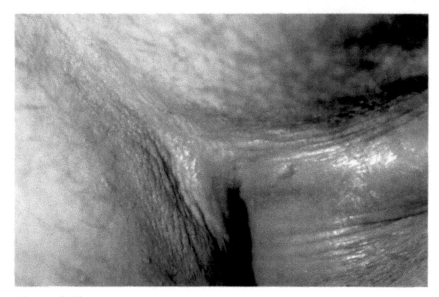

Figure 2.19

Tinea cruris—differential diagnosis: seborrhoeic dermatitis. Seborrhoeic dermatitis is not unusual in the inguinal region. The fold may be macerated to form fissures. There is no peripheral active border as in fungal infection. Often the skin of the scrotum is also involved. As in fungal infection, inguinal seborrhoeic dermatitis is predominantly a male disorder.

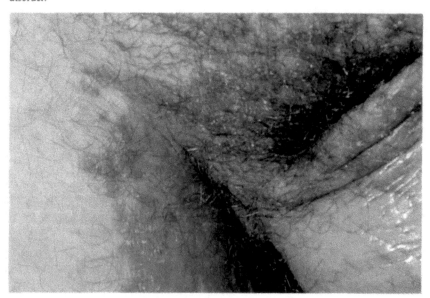

Figure 2.20

Tinea cruris—differential diagnosis: psoriasis. In widespread psoriasis the inguinal region may be severely affected. The symptoms may resemble seborrhoeic dermatitis. Psoriatic lesions in other skin areas help in the differential diagnosis.

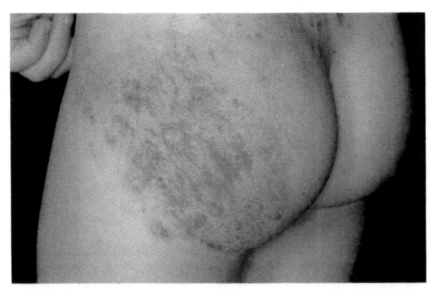

a

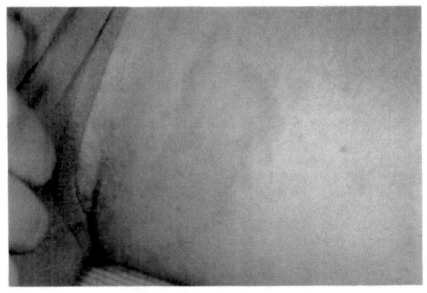

b

Figure 2.21

Tinea cruris—differential diagnosis: atopic eczema. (a) In children fungal infection is less common than atopic dermatitis. The itchy gluteal atopic dermatitis may be scratched and secondarily infected by bacteria, most typically staphylococci. (b) Atopic dermatitis in a young boy at the inner aspect of the leg. Lesions with a more active peripheral region may simulate ringworm. Symptoms and signs in other skin areas, and negative mycology, help in the diagnosis. In children fungal infection in this location is very uncommon.

45

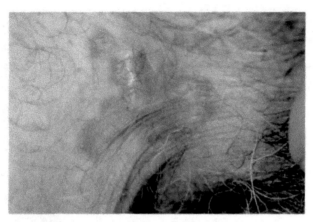

Figure 2.22

Tinea cruris—differential diagnosis: inguinal lichen planus. Lichen planus only rarely affects skin folds, as here in the inguinal region. The violaceous edge surrounds the reddish central area. The same features may also be found in the axillary region and on the sides of the lower neck. The typical colour, and negative mycology, differentiates lichen planus from fungal disease.

Tinea manuum

The hand may be affected (Figures 2.23–2.25) by dermatophyte fungal infection (tinea manuum), but it is quite rare for the hands to be affected alone, the feet typically being the main site. Both feet and one hand may show concurrent infection (the two feet–one-hand syndrome).

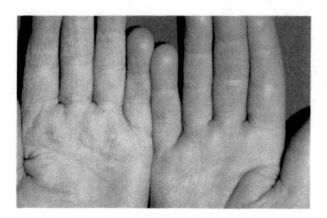

Figure 2.23

Tinea manuum—one-hand tinea. Palmar mycosis is predominantly unilateral. The symptoms are generally mild, with 'sharply' marginated lesions. Occasionally, fungal pustules may develop. The causative agent is almost invariably T. rubrum, which has generally caused the plantar (and nail) mycosis before the appearance of hand symptoms.

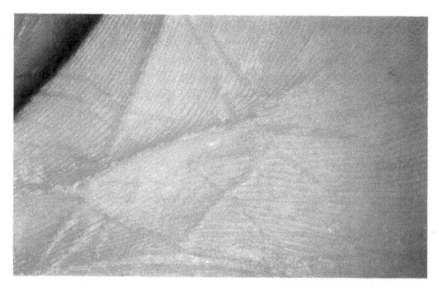

Figure 2.24
Tinea manuum—slight scaling.

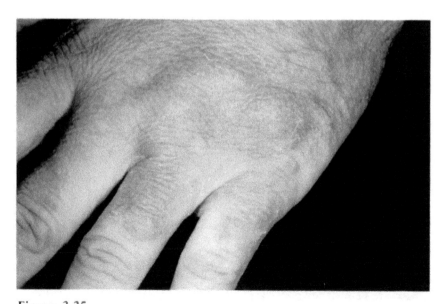

Figure 2.25
Tinea manuum—dorsal surface also affected. An unusual form of T. rubrum *infection on the dorsum of the hand. The affected area is violaceous, oedematous and slightly scaling. This male patient also suffers from unilateral (same-side) palmar and bilateral plantar tinea. Therapy with terbinafine 250 mg once daily for 14 days was successful.*

47

Tinea corporis (tinea circinata, ringworm)

These fungal infections (Figures 2.26–2.32) involve the glabrous skin and produce lesions ranging from vesicles through scaling eczematous lesions to deep granulomata. Though found universally, these infections occur more commonly in tropical to temperate climates.

Clinical features

The most common form is the annular erythematous, papulosquamous lesion. Rings of papules with central healing are grouped in clusters. Some lesions, through lack of spontaneous healing, spread chronically to form large scaling plaques.

Majocchi's granuloma is essentially a granulomatous folliculitis and perifolliculitis; a typical site is at the wrist under the watch-strap.

With careful treatment, tinea corporis ringworm responds to treatment within approximately 2 weeks. Relapse is rare.

Some conditions that mimic tinea corporis are shown in Figures 2.33–2.39.

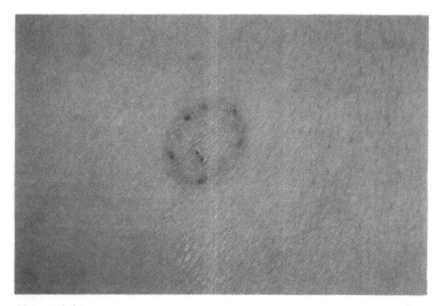

Figure 2.26

Tinea corporis—ringworm. The diameter of the ringworm lesion is approximately 3 cm. The infection is caused by T. rubrum. *On the basis of the clinical picture alone, infection caused by, for example,* M. canis *cannot be excluded.*

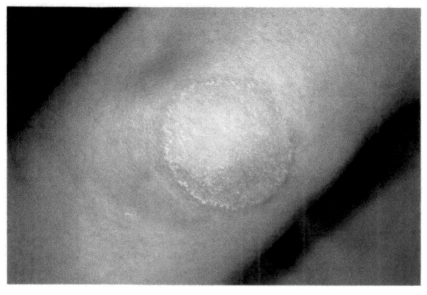

Figure 2.27
Tinea corporis—ringworm at the elbow region. The active peripheral rim differentiates it from any psoriatic lesion, which is more common at this site. This infection was caused by T. mentagrophytes *transmitted by a pet guinea-pig.*

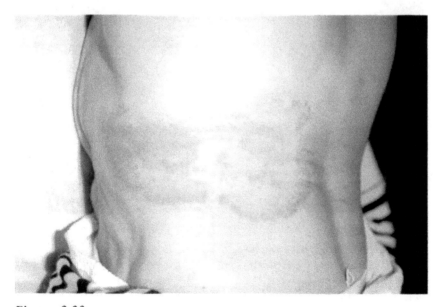

Figure 2.28
Tinea corporis —ringworm. A large ringworm on the left side of the thoracic skin. The causative dermatophyte is T. mentagrophytes. *The patient also had tinea in the genital region and lower legs.*

49

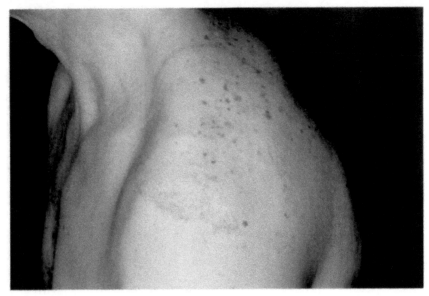

Figure 2.29

Tinea corporis—ringworm. A large patch of ringworm on the left shoulder. The disease was caused by T. mentagrophytes. *If localised, tinea corporis can be treated with topical agents; in more widespread cases systemic therapy is preferred.*

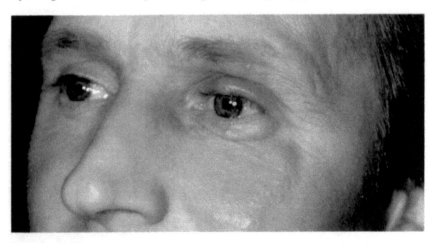

Figure 2.30

Tinea corporis—tinea faciei. Here, the left eyelid is affected. This young farmer also had a ringworm in front of the ankle. T. mentagrophytes *dermatophyte was transmitted from cattle. Because of the involvement of the eyelid, oral antifungal therapy was necessary.*

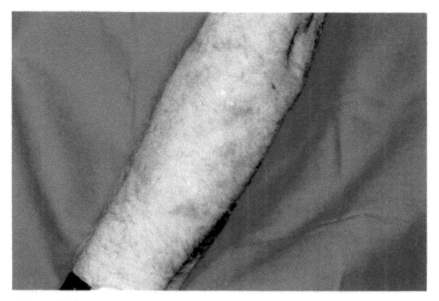

Figure 2.31

Tinea corporis—upper arm. Widespread ringworm on the arm with many fungal pustules in the affected area. The infection is caused by T. rubrum. *Therapy with terbinafine 250 mg once daily for 14 days was effective.*

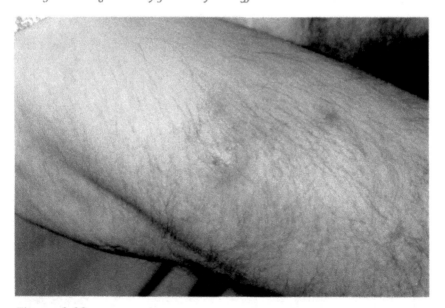

Figure 2.32

Tinea corporis—upper arm; small pustules. Follicular inflammation, and even focal pustules on a limited area of the arm, may be caused by T. rubrum. *The differential diagnosis is often clinically difficult, but fungal elements in a KOH preparation and fungal culture confirm the diagnosis. Oral therapy with terbinafine 250 mg once daily for 14 days healed the lesions.*

51

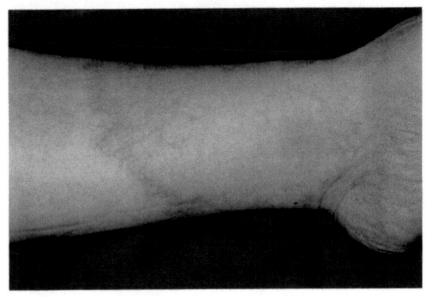

Figure 2.33
Tinea corporis—differential diagnosis: erythema migrans, an early phase skin symptom of borrelial infection. The erythematous edge is less conspicuous than in fungal infection, and scaling is unusual.

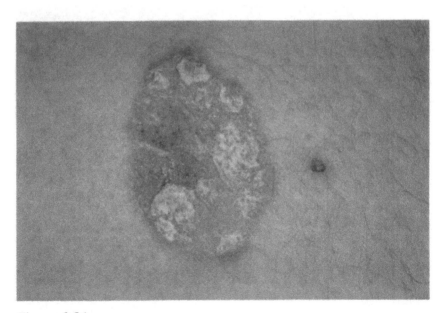

Figure 2.34
Tinea corporis—differential diagnosis: psoriasis.

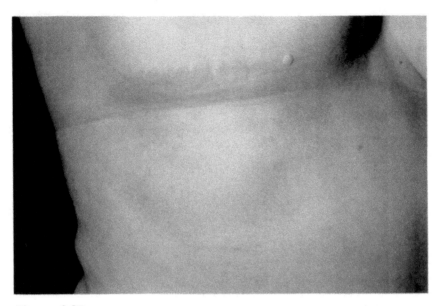

Figure 2.35
Tinea corporis—differential diagnosis: localised scleroderma.

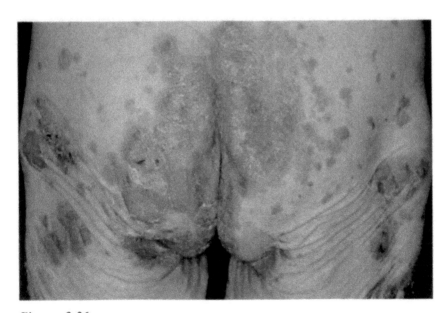

Figure 2.36
Tinea corporis—differential diagnosis: glucagonoma syndrome.

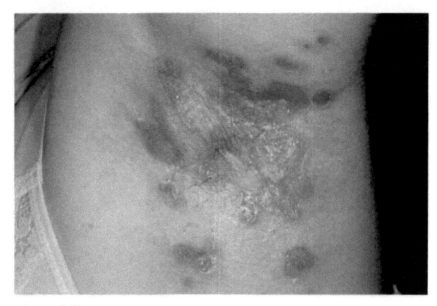

Figure 2.37
Tinea corporis—differential diagnosis: axillary impetigo.

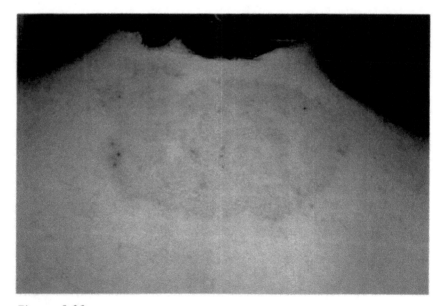

Figure 2.38
Tinea corporis—differential diagnosis: seborrhoeic dermatitis.

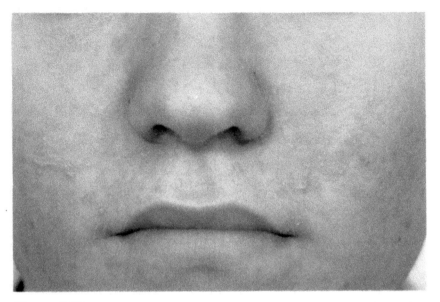

Figure 2.39
Tinea corporis—differential diagnosis: facial seborrhoeic dermatitis.

Tinea barbae (tinea sycosis; tinea faciei)

Tinea barbae *cum* faciei (Figures 2.40–2.43) is a chronic infection of the areas of the face and neck that have large hair follicles. It is associated with various species of *Trichophyton* and occasionally with *Microsporum canis*.

It mainly occurs in Europe and the USA, particularly in farming areas. The disease most frequently affects agricultural workers who come into contact with farm animals, mainly cattle.

Clinical features

The disease produces a superficial crusted lesion. Pustular folliculitis with or without broken hairs may be observed. Deep, nodular, suppurative lesions, nodular thickening and kerion-type swelling may also be noted.

Prognosis is good as the infection responds to oral griseofulvin, terbinafine and itraconazole in particular. Relapse or recurrence is rare.

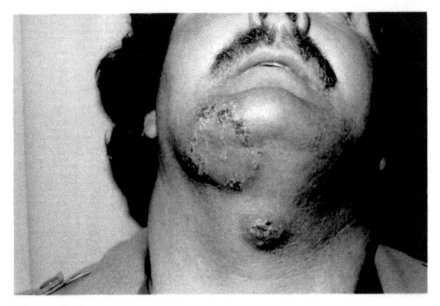

Figure 2.40
Tinea barbae—multiple erythematous lesions.

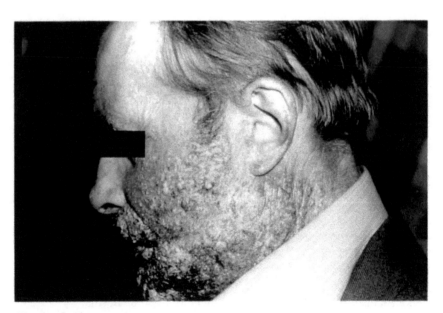

Figure 2.41
Tinea barbae—severe diffuse beard involvement.

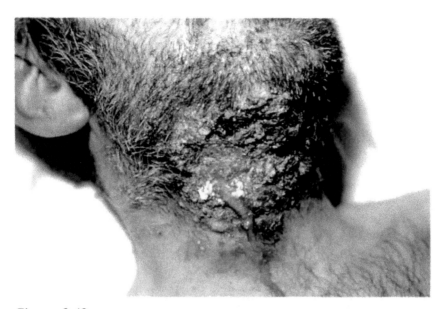

Figure 2.42
Tinea barbae—pseudoabscess appearance.

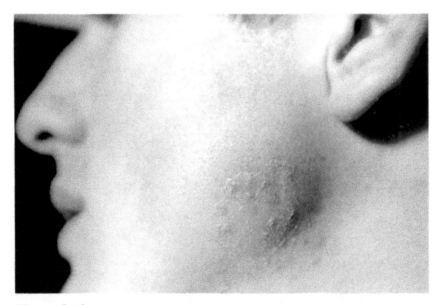

Figure 2.43
Tinea facei—focal lesion with follicular lesions in evidence.

Tinea capitis

Tinea capitis (Figures 2.44–2.52) is ringworm of the scalp. The basic feature of the infection is invasion of the hair shafts by dermatophyte fungi.

Most species of dermatophytes are capable of invading the hair, but some species, such as *Microsporum audouinii*, *Trichophyton schoenleinii* and *T. violaceum*, have a particular predilection for the hair shaft.

The species of dermatophyte fungus most likely to cause tinea capitis vary from country to country and often from region to region. In any given location the species may change with time, particularly as new organisms are introduced by immigration. It is of interest that, in tinea capitis, anthropophilic species predominate. In recent years there has been an increase in *M. canis* as the dominant organism of infection in Europe, and a spread of *T. tonsurans* in urban communities in Europe and the USA.

The conidia of the ringworm fungi that cause tinea capitis can be demonstrated in the atmosphere close to the scalp of patients with the condition. It is highly likely that scalp hair acts as a trapping device, possibly enhanced by electrostatic forces. It is known that contamination of hair without any clinical signs may occur among classmates of children with tinea capitis. It has also been demonstrated that, if actual hair infection is to occur, the stratum corneum of the scalp skin must first be invaded. Trauma assists inoculation.

There are several types of hair invasion that should be noted.

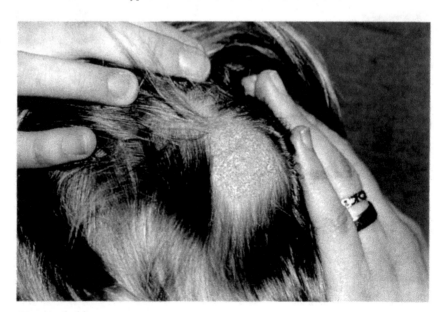

Figure 2.44
Tinea capitis—relatively uninflamed scalp ringworm due to M. canis *—from a dog or cat.*

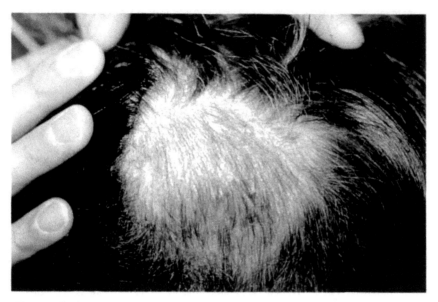

Figure 2.45
Tinea capitis—showing hair breakage and some inflammation.

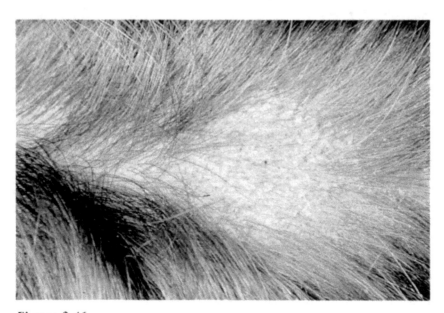

Figure 2.46
Tinea capitis—a relatively uninflamed scalp ringworm due to T. verrucosum.

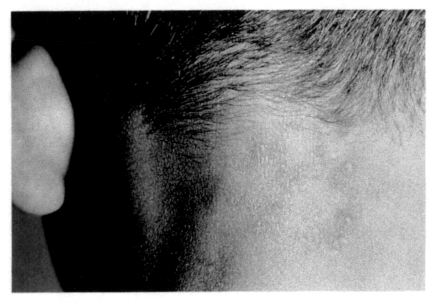

Figure 2.47
Tinea capitis—scalp margin and neck ringworm due to T. verrucosum.

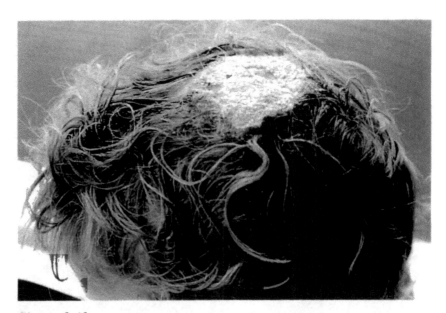

Figure 2.48
Tinea capitis, kerion type—pseudoabscess appearance.

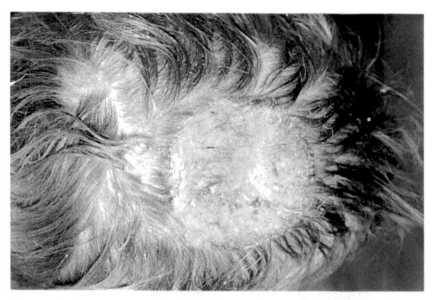

Figure 2.49
Tinea capitis, kerion type—a flatter lesion without crusting or purulent appearance.

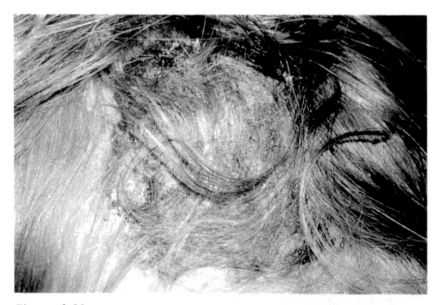

Figure 2.50
Tinea capitis, kerion type—severely crusting lesion.

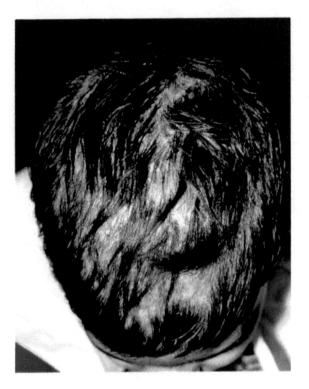

Figure 2.51
Tinea capitis, favus type (due to T. schoenleinii). Thick yellow scales occur in the early stages.

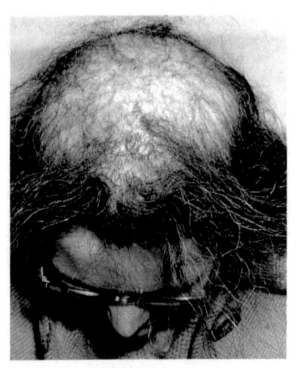

Figure 2.52
Tinea capitis, favus type (due to T. schoenleinii). Diffuse scarring with little or no scaling may be evident in late stages.

Microsporum type

In *small-spored ectothrix* (e.g. *M. canis*), the hair shaft is invaded to the mid-follicle. Intrafollicular hyphae continue to grow inwards towards the bulb of the hair. Secondary extrapiliary hyphae burst out and grow in a tortuous manner over the surface of the hair shaft. Under Wood's ultraviolet light, a bluish-green fluorescence is characteristically observed.

Trichophyton type

In *large-spored ectothrix* (*in chains*) (e.g. *T. verrucosum*) the arthrospores are spherical and arranged in straight chains. Again, they are confined to the outer surface of the hair shaft. There is no fluorescence.

In *endothrix* (e.g. *T. tonsurans*), intrapilary hyphae fragment into arthrospores, which are entirely within the hair shaft. Hair thus affected is fragile and breaks off close to the scalp surface. This type is non-fluorescent.

In the *favic type* (e.g. *T. schoenleinii*), broad hyphae and air spaces are seen in the hair shaft but arthrospores are always absent. The affected hair is less damaged than in the other types of the invasion and may continue to grow to considerable lengths. Greenish-grey fluorescence is present.

Clinical features

The clinical appearance of ringworm of the scalp is quite variable, depending on the type of hair invasion, the level of host resistance and the degree of inflammatory host response. Its appearance, therefore, may vary from a few dull grey broken-off hairs (with a little scaling detectable only on careful inspection) to a severe, painful inflammatory mass covering most of the scalp. In all types the main features are partial hair loss with inflammation to some degree. It is useful to recognize several basic clinical pictures.

Small-spored ectothrix infections

In *M. audouinii* and *M. ferrugineum* infections, the basic lesions are patches of partial alopecia that are often circular in shape. These patches have broken-off hairs that are a dull grey colour as a result of their coating of arthrospores. Inflammation is minor but fine scaling is characteristic—usually with a fairly distinct margin. There may be several such patches. In *M. canis* infection, there is more inflammatory change. In infection caused by all these species, a green

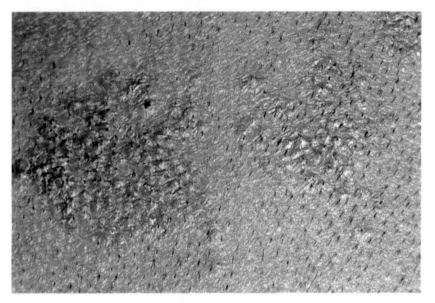

Figure 2.53
'Black dot' endothrix tinea capitis in an Australian Aborigine showing numerous broken-off infected hairs and pustular lesions of the scalp.

fluorescence under Wood's ultraviolet light is usual, but non-fluorescent cases have been reported. Children are affected more frequently than adults.

Kerion

The most severe pattern of reaction is known as a kerion. This is a painful inflammatory mass in which such hairs as remain are loose. Follicles may be seen discharging pus, there may be sinus formation and, on rare occasions, mycetoma-like grains may be found. Thick crusting with matting of adjacent hairs is common. The area affected may be limited, but multiple plaques are not rare and occasionally a large confluent lesion may involve much of the scalp. Regional lymphadenopathy is common. Although this violent reaction is usually caused by one of the zoophilic species, typically *T. verrucosum* or *T. mentagrophytes*, occasionally a geophilic organism is isolated and anthropophilic infections that have been relatively inactive for weeks may suddenly become inflammatory. These develop kerions if there is a high degree of hypersensitivity. The possibility that a secondary bacterial infection may be playing some part should not be ignored. In such cases, a swab should be sent to the bacterial laboratory

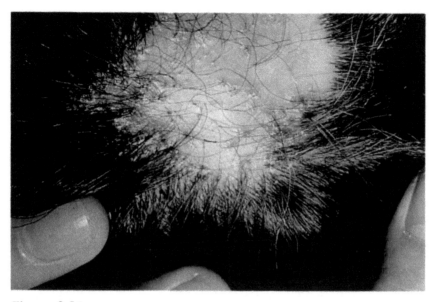

Figure 2.54
Favus of the scalp showing extensive hair loss and numerous small scutula. T. schoenleinii was isolated.

in addition to hairs plucked for mycology. If treatment is instituted without undue delay, healing should occur without residual scarring.

Endothrix infections

In *T. tonsurans* and *T. violaceum* infections, a relatively non-inflammatory type of patchy baldness occurs. The formation of black dots (swollen hair shafts) as the affected hair breaks at the surface of the scalp is a classical sign in this condition, but such findings may not be very conspicuous (Figure 2.53). The patches, which are usually multiple, may show minimal scaling. They are commonly angular in outline rather than round. A low-grade folliculitis is often seen, and sometimes a kerion may develop.

Favus

Infection with *T. schoenleinii* is seen sporadically in many countries. The classical picture of tinea capitis as a result of this organism is the presence of yellowish, cup-shaped crusts known as scutula (Figure 2.54). Each scutulum develops around a hair, which pierces it centrally. Adjacent crusts enlarge to become confluent, forming a mass of yellow crusting. Extensive patchy hair loss with cicatricial alopecia and atrophy among patches of normal hair may be found in long-standing cases. Here, much of the hair loss is irreversible as a result of the destruction of the bulge area of the hair follicle. Although the initial infection probably occurs in childhood in nearly all cases, it shows little if any tendency to clear spontaneously at puberty, particularly in women. Families with several generations of affected offspring have been well documented.

Several conditions may mimic scalp fungal infections. Some commoner examples are shown in Figures 2.55–2.62.

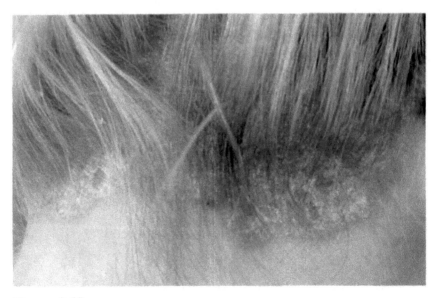

Figure 2.55
Tinea capitas—differential diagnosis: scalp psoriasis. The scale is typically more obvious than fungal disease and is usually silvery.

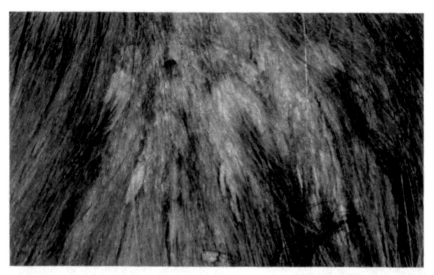

Figure 2.56

Tinea capitis—differential diagnosis: pityriasis amiantacea. Thick, asbestos-like, soft hyperkeratosis, often in localised areas of the scalp, is a relatively common phenomenon. It is sometimes a feature of seborrhoeic dermatitis but may be a symptom of atopic dermatitis or psoriasis. The hair shafts may be secondarily broken, making differentiation from tinea capitis more difficult. Mycological specimens should be taken.

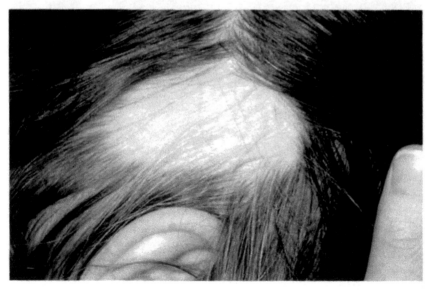

Figure 2.57

Tinea capitis—differential diagnosis: alopecia areata.

67

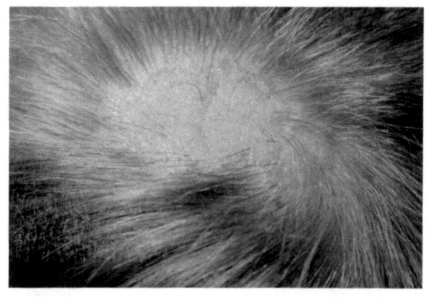

Figure 2.58
Tinea capitis—differential diagnosis: naevus sebaceus. The best differential diagnostic feature of this hamartoma is its presence from birth. The surface may be slightly verrucous. There are no hairs.

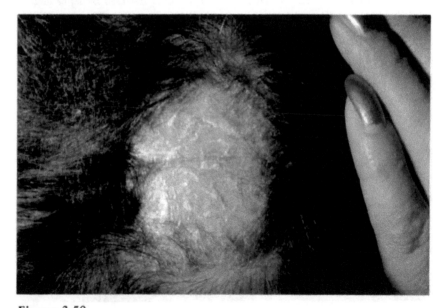

Figure 2.59
Tinea capitis—differential diagnosis: discoid lupus erythematosus. In the early phase this reddish, slowly enlarging patch with associated hair loss may be difficult to differentiate from tinea capitis. The histopathological features are mostly diagnostic, and mycology is negative.

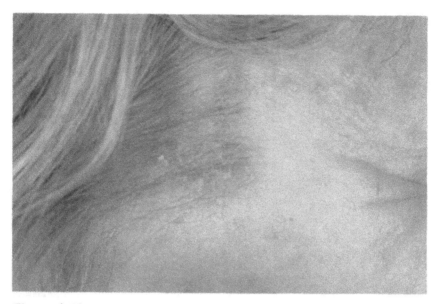

Figure 2.60

Tinea capitis—differential diagnosis: seborrhoeic dermatitis.

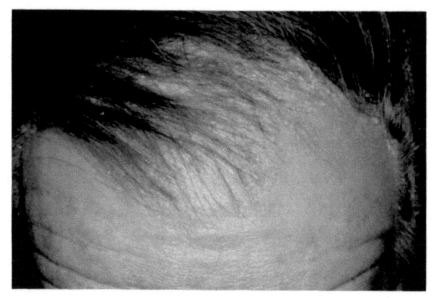

Figure 2.61

Tinea capitis—differential diagnosis: seborrhoeic dermatitis. The frontal hair line is one of the major sites of seborrhoeic dermatitis. No damage to the hair shafts is found. Differential diagnosis from psoriasis may be difficult without also examining other skin areas.

69

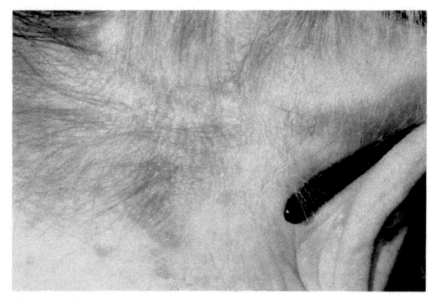

Figure 2.62
Tinea capitis—differential diagnosis: lichen planus.

Tinea nigra

Tinea nigra (Figures 2.63 and 2.64) is a superficial fungal infection of skin characterized by brown to black macules that usually occur on the palmar aspects of the hands and, occasionally, on the plantar and other surfaces of the skin. Lesions are non-inflammatory and non-scaling. The familial spread of infection has been reported. Infections have been reported worldwide, but are more common in the tropical regions of Central and South America, Africa, southeast Asia and Australia. The causative agent is *Phaeoannellomyces (Exophiala) werneckii*, which is a common saprophytic fungus believed to occur in soil, compost, humus and on wood in humid tropical and subtropical regions.

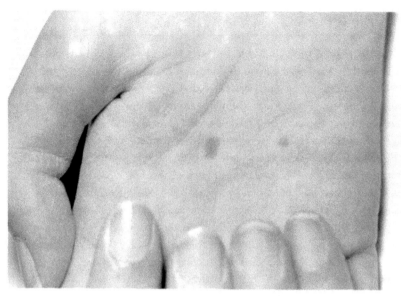

Figure 2.63

Tinea nigra (synonyms: pityriasis nigra; tinea nigra palmaris; keratomycosis nigricans palmaris) is due to P. werneckii. *It is usually asymptomatic, presenting as a pigmented, non-scaly patch.*

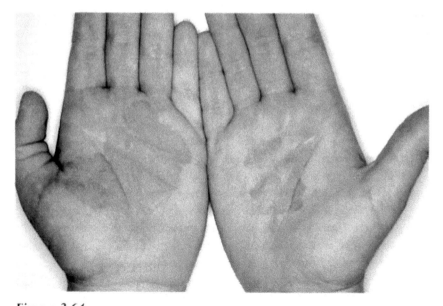

Figure 2.64

Typical brown to black, non-scaling macules on the palmar aspect of the hands. There is no inflammatory reaction.

71

Black piedra

The superficial fungal infection due to *Piedra hortae* and called black piedra is characterized by hard, black nodules that cling firmly to the affected hair shaft. *Piedra* ('stone' in Spanish) describes these gritty, adherent concretions, which are difficult to scrape off. Combing affected hairs with a metal comb is said to produce a characteristic rattling sound. Normal hair intervenes between the nodules and is not significantly weakened. As a result, nodules may be present throughout the length of the hair.

Transmission may be from person to person, through close contact or through shared combs. Epidemics among schoolchildren have occurred in Thailand and in Puerto Rico. In South America, black piedra is more common after puberty and in those with long hair, whether male or female.

Infection is asymptomatic, and alopecia does not occur. The brown to black nodules may encircle the hair shaft. The concretions may achieve 1.5 mm in length, attaching via hyphae to the superficial cortex.

Wood's ultraviolet light examination is negative, but light microscopy reveals compact, dark, thick-walled septate hyphae in an organized geometric mass. Within the mature nodule, paler loculi or asci appear like honeycombs.

White piedra may occur concurrently with black piedra.

White piedra

The offending yeast of this infection is named *Trichosporon beigelii* (although the name *Trichosporon cutaneum* has also been used). *Trichosporon* may be recovered in abundance from the environment, as well as from mammals and from human sputum, stools and skin, even in the absence of clinical disease.

Cases of white piedra are sporadic in tropical and temperate climates, but reports from very cold climates (Scandinavia) have been published.

The infection, which may be subclinical and asymptomatic or obvious and irritating, is manifested by whitish, soft, nodular concretions of *T. beigelii* that cling to the hair shafts of the scalp, face, axillae or perigenital area, either discretely or coalesced into a sheath. The fusiform masses can be scraped off—unlike the hard, dark ovoids in black piedra. The hair shaft is weakened by the fungal invasion of the cortex, so that 'split end' trichorrhexis nodosa and partial alopecia may result. The infection of genital hairs is now thought to be the most common manifestation, although concurrent infection of multiple sites can occur. In the scalp, pruritus may be the presenting complaint.

Diagnosis

The nodules are composed of closely packed, septate hyphae and blastoconidia in a dense geometric array. The arthroconidia are uniformly nearly round. Elevation of the hair cuticle is often visible within the nodule. The fungal mass is much paler than that seen in black piedra, and loculis are absent. Corynebacteria frequently accompany the fungal nodules and may emit a faint yellowish glow under Wood's ultraviolet light. *Trichosporon* does not fluoresce. Clinically, white piedra can be almost impossible to distinguish from trichomycosis axillaris or pubis. It does not, however, cause staining of the clothes or emit a foul odour. Other concretions of the hair shaft that must be excluded are the same as those listed for black piedra.

Cutaneous candidiasis

Candidiasis is a primary or secondary mycotic infection caused by members of the genus *Candida*. The clinical manifestations may be acute, subacute or chronic to episodic. Involvement may be localised to the mouth, throat, skin, scalp, vagina, fingers, nails, bronchi, lungs or the gastrointestinal tract, or become systemic as in septicaemia, endocarditis and meningitis. In healthy individuals, *Candida* infections are usually the result of impaired epithelial barrier functions and they occur in all age groups but are most common in the newborn and the elderly. They usually remain superficial and respond readily to treatment. Systemic candidiasis is usually seen in patients with cell-mediated immune deficiency, and those receiving aggressive cancer treatment or other immunosuppressive therapy.

Several species of *Candida* may be aetiological agents (see Chapter 1), most commonly, *Candida albicans*. All are ubiquitous and occur naturally on humans, especially *C. albicans*, which is recognised as a commensal of the gastrointestinal tract.

Oropharyngeal candidiasis

(Including thrush, glossitis, stomatitis and angular cheilitis.)

Acute oral candidiasis (Figures 2.65–2.68) is rarely seen in healthy adults but may occur in up to 5% of newborn infants and 10% of the elderly. However, it is often associated with severe immunological impairment due to diabetes mellitus, leukaemia, lymphoma, malignancy, neutropenia and HIV infection, where it presents as a predictor of clinical progression to AIDS. The

73

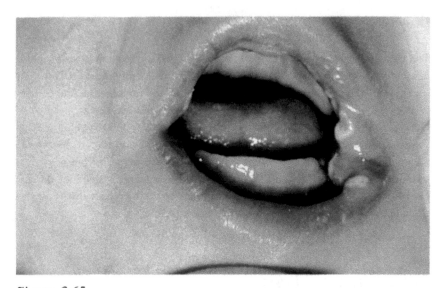

Figure 2.65

Oral candidiasis in an infant showing characteristic patches of a creamy-white to grey pseudomembrane composed of blastoconidia and pseudohyphae of C. albicans. The mouth of normal newborn infants has a low pH, which may promote the proliferation of C. albicans. The infections are usually acquired during the birth process from mothers who had vaginal thrush during pregnancy. Clinical symptoms may persist until a balanced oral flora has been established.

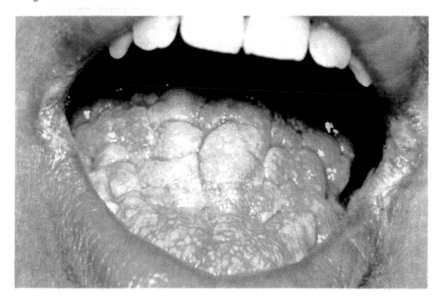

Figure 2.66

Chronic oral candidiasis of the tongue and mouth corners (angular cheilitis) in an adult with underlying immune deficiency. The characteristic white pseudomembrane is composed of the cells and pseudohyphae of C. albicans.

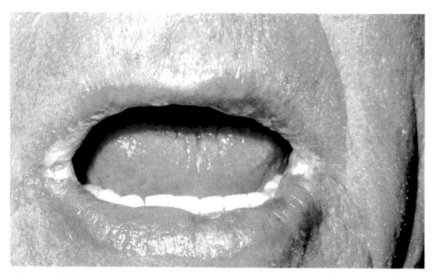

Figure 2.67
Angular cheilitis—intertrigo and fissuring caused by maceration of the corners of the mouth are frequently complicated by chronic infection with C. albicans. There are white pseudomembrane-like colonies in the mouth corners of this adult patient.

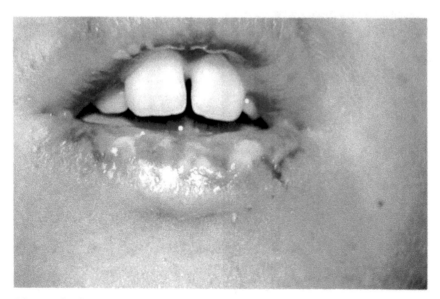

Figure 2.68
Solar cheilitis in a young boy showing colonisation of the lip by C. albicans.

use of broad-spectrum antibiotics, corticosteroids, cytotoxic drugs and radiation therapy is also a predisposing factor. Clinically, white plaques that resemble milk curd form on the buccal mucosa and, less commonly, on the tongue, gums, palate or pharynx. Symptoms may be absent or include burning or dryness of the mouth, loss of taste and pain on swallowing.

Cutaneous candidiasis

(Including intertrigo types, diaper candidiasis, paronychia and onychomycosis (see also Chapter 3) (Figures 2.69–2.79).)

Intertriginous candidiasis is most commonly seen in the axillae, groin, inter- and submammary folds, intergluteal folds, interdigital spaces and umbilicus. Moisture, heat, friction and maceration of the skin are the principal predisposing factors in the normal patient. However, obesity, diabetes mellitus, warm-water immersion or occlusion of the skin and the use of broad-spectrum antibiotics are additional factors. Lesions consist of a moist, macular erythematous rash with typical satellite lesions present on the surrounding healthy skin.

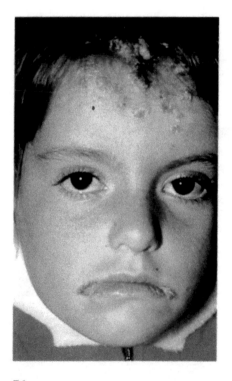

Figure 2.69
Candida granuloma of the forehead and angular cheilitis of the mouth in a young girl with chronic mucocutaneous candidiasis. There are thick crusted lesions of the scalp and forehead. C. albicans *was isolated.*

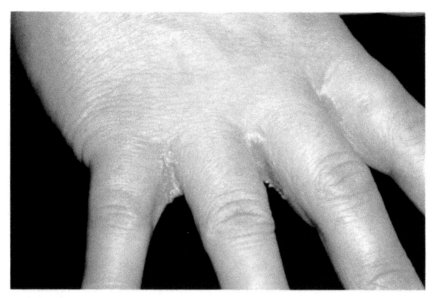

Figure 2.70

Interdigital candidiasis of the hands may develop particularly in persons whose hands are subject to continuing wetting, especially with sugar solutions or through contact with flour. C. albicans *was isolated.*

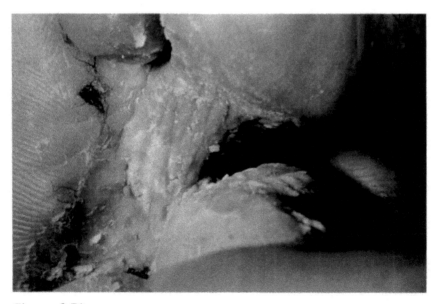

Figure 2.71

Interdigital candidiasis of the feet explains 1% of cases of 'athletes foot' and must be distinguished from tinea pedis caused by dermatophytes. C. albicans *was isolated.*

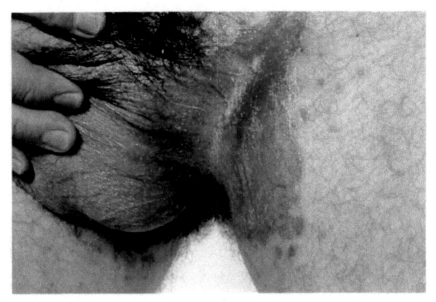

Figure 2.72
Intertriginous or flexural candidiasis of the groin may also mimic tinea cruris caused by
a dermatophyte. There are erythematous scaling lesions with a distinctive border and
several small satellite lesions. C. albicans was isolated.

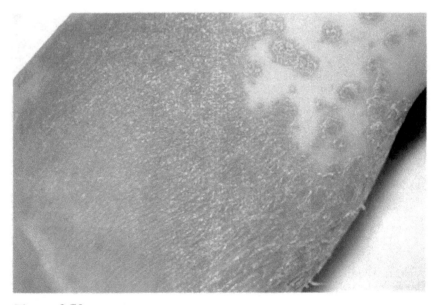

Figure 2.73
Intertriginous or flexural candidiasis behind the knee showing an extensive erythematous
scaling lesion and several smaller satellite lesions caused by C. albicans.

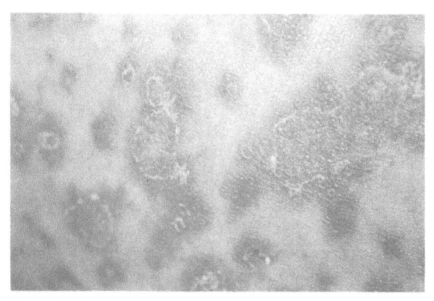

Figure 2.74
Satellite lesions of cutaneous candidiasis showing typical scale collars. C. albicans *was isolated. The presence of satellite lesions usually differentiates candidiasis from dermatophytosis.*

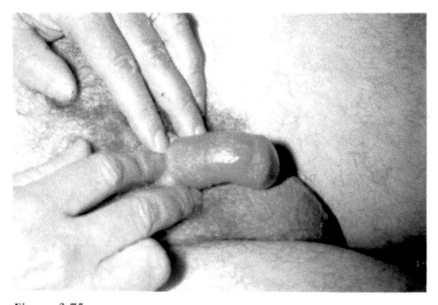

Figure 2.75
Candidiasis of the penis (balanitis) caused by C. albicans.

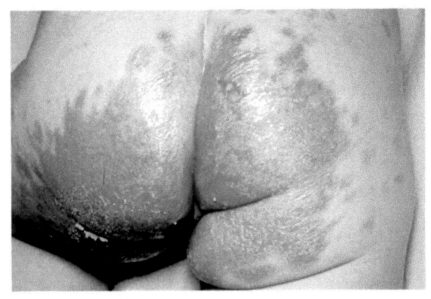

Figure 2.76

Superficial candidiasis in an infant (nappy rash) secondary to seborrhoeic dermatitis. This usually occurs under the unhygienic conditions of chronic dampness and irregularly changed, unclean nappies. In some cases this condition may spread to the axillae, face, conjunctiva and other areas (see Figure 2.77).

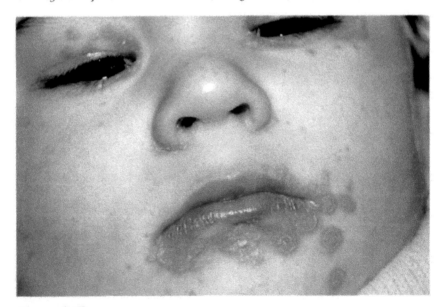

Figure 2.77

A young infant with chronic superficial candidiasis showing spread to the mouth area and conjunctiva. The erythematous scaling lesions have well marginated borders and the small satellite lesions on the chin show the typical collar of scaling. C. albicans was isolated.

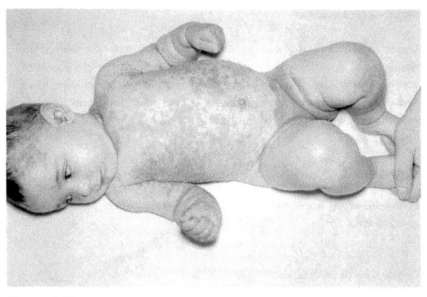

Figure 2.78
Generalized candidiasis in a young infant secondary to seborrhoeic dermatitis caused by
C. albicans. Here there is a particular involvement of the body creases (e.g. groin,
axillae, neck and cubital fossae) and multiple small satellite lesions.

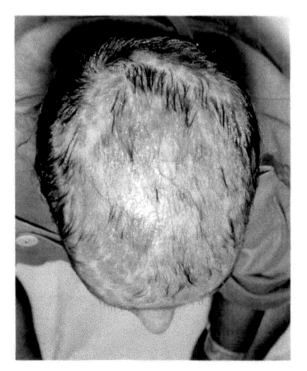

Figure 2.79
Chronic candidiasis of
the scalp in a child with
an underlying immune
deficiency caused by C.
albicans.

81

Diaper napkin candidiasis

Diaper napkin candidiasis is common in infants living under the unhygienic conditions of chronic moisture and local skin maceration that are associated with ammonitic irritation due to irregularly changed, unclean diapers. Once again, characteristic erythematous lesions with erosions and satellite pustules are produced, with prominent involvement of the skin folds and creases.

Paronychia

Paronychia of the finger nails may develop in persons whose hands are subject to continuous wetting (see Chapter 3).

Chronic Candida onychomycosis

Chronic *Candida* onychomycosis often causes the complete destruction of nail tissue (see Chapter 3).

Vulvovaginal candidiasis

Vulvovaginal candidiasis is a common condition in women, often associated with the use of broad-spectrum antibiotics, the third trimester of pregnancy, low vaginal pH and diabetes mellitus. Sexual activity and oral contraception may also be contributing factors, and infections may extend to include the perineum, the vulva and the entire inguinal area. Chronic refractory vaginal candidiasis, associated with oral candidiasis, may also be a presentation of HIV infection or AIDS. Symptoms include intense vulval pruritus, burning, erythema and dyspareunia associated with a creamy-white, curd-like discharge.

Balanitis

In cases of balanitis, diabetes mellitus should be excluded and the sexual partner should be investigated for vulvovaginitis. The symptoms include erythema, pruritus and vesiculopustules on the glan penis or prepuce. Infections are more commonly seen in uncircumcised men, and poor hygiene may also be a contributing factor.

Malassezia infections

Pityriasis (tinea) versicolor

Pityriasis versicolor (Figures 2.80–2.82) is a chronic, superficial fungal disease of the skin characterised by well demarcated white, pink, fawn or brownish lesions, often coalescing, and covered with thin furfuraceous scales. The colour varies according to the normal pigmentation of the patient, exposure of the area to sunlight and the severity of the disease. Lesions occur on the trunk, shoulders and arms and rarely on the neck and face, and fluoresce a pale greenish colour under Wood's ultraviolet light. Young adults are affected most often, but the disease may occur in childhood and old age. The causative agent is *Malassezia furfur* (*Pityrosporum orbiculare*), a lipophilic yeast living on the skin as part of the normal flora. The diagnosis may be confirmed in most cases by direct microscopic examination of skin scrapings mounted in 10% KOH with Parker ink to show the characteristic spherical yeast cells and short, pseudohyphal elements typical of the fungus. Culture is unnecessary as direct microscopy is diagnostic.

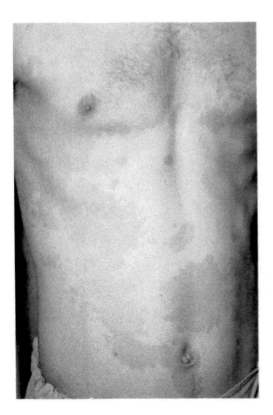

Figure 2.80
Pityriasis versicolor—brown macule form. Pityriasis versicolor is a patchy, macular eruption usually with very little in the way of symptoms. The colour may vary from reddish-brown to grey or white. After treatment the lesions tend to be white, especially during or immediately after summer, because the lesional skin temporarily loses its normal pigment.

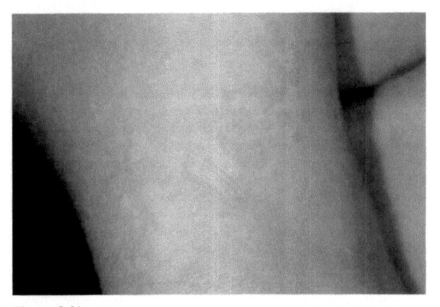

Figure 2.81
Pityriasis versicolor—reddish variant.

Figure 2.82
Pityriasis versicolor—whitish patch.

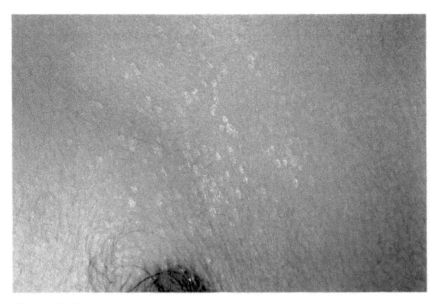

Figure 2.83

Follicular pityriasis (seborrhoeic folliculitis)—lesions are visible around the hair follicles and sebaceous glands. This is a more severe form of the disease.

Pityrosporum ('seborrhoeic') folliculitis

Pityrosporum folliculitis is characterised by follicular papules and pustules localised to the back, chest and upper arms (Figure 2.83), sometimes the neck, and more seldom the face. These are itchy and often appear after sun exposure. Scrapings or biopsy specimens show numerous yeasts occluding the mouths of the infected follicles.

Seborrhoeic dermatitis and pityriasis capitis (dandruff)

Current evidence suggests *M. furfur*, combined with multifactorial host factors, is also the direct cause of seborrhoeic dermatitis, with dandruff being the mildest manifestation. Host factors include genetic predisposition, neurologically mediated factors, changes in quantity and composition of sebum (increase in wax esters and a shift from triglycerides to shorter fatty acid chains), increase in alkalinity of skin (due to eccrine sweating) and external local factors such as occlusion. Patients with neurological diseases (such as Parkinson's disease) and those with AIDS are commonly affected. Clinical manifestations are characterised by erythema and scaling in areas with a rich supply of sebaceous glands, i.e. the scalp, face, eyebrows, ears and upper trunk. Lesions are red and covered with greasy scales. Itching is common in the scalp. The clinical features are typical and skin scrapings for a laboratory diagnosis are unnecessary.

3 NAILS (ONYCHOMYCOSIS): CLINICAL ASPECTS

Onychomycosis is the infection of the nail by fungi. Most cases of onychomycosis result from dermatophytic invasion of the nail. Onychomycosis as a result of non-dermatophytic moulds or yeast is relatively rare (Figure 3.1).

The normal intact nail apparatus is so well designed (in functional anatomical terms) that it can generally resist external influences, such as fungal invasion. Nails will resist primary invasion by organisms unless the body's immunosuppression system is present due to drugs or disease. Therefore the clinician obtaining positive microscopy or culture should ask why the organism has become established.

Onychomycosis due to dermatophytes

(See Figures 3.2–3.19.) Three different routes of nail invasion by dermatophytic fungi have been described:

1) Distal and lateral subungual onychomycosis (DLSO).
2) Proximal subungual onychomycosis (PSO).
3) White superficial onychomycosis (WSO).

More recently, a fourth route of invasion of the nail matrix by dermatophytes has been described: endonyx onychomycosis (EO).

In distal and lateral subungual onychomycosis (DLSO) the most common route of invasion—dermatophytes reach the nail bed via the hyponychium. The skin on the soles of the feet is the primary site of infection, and plantar scaling is usually associated with this type of onychomycosis. The distal nail bed reacts to dermatophyte invasion by becoming somewhat inflamed and hyperkeratotic. This results in subungual hyperkeratosis, the typical sign of DLSO. Eventually, the nail plate separates from the nail bed, which results in onycholysis. The total destruction of the entire thickness of the nail plate

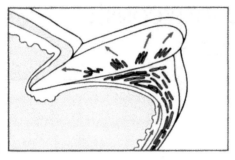

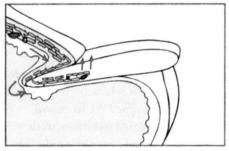

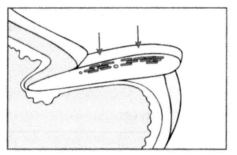

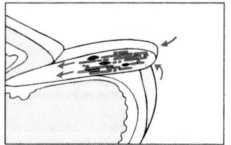

Figure 3.1
Onychomycosis—the arrows show the directions of invasion.
(a) Distal and lateral subungual onychomycosis (DLSO).
(b) Proximal subungual onychomycosis (PSO). (c) White superficial onychomycosis (WSO).
(d) Endonyx onychomycosis (EO).

Reproduced from Dawber R, Bristow I, Mooney J (1996) The Foot: Problems in Podiatry and Dermatology (Martin Dunitz: London).

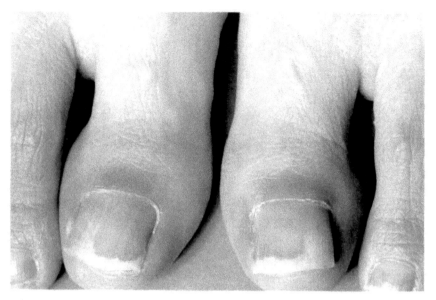

Figure 3.2
Tinea unguium—early-stage involvement of the great toenails showing onycholysis.

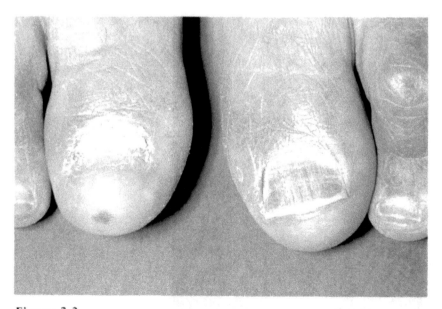

Figure 3.3
Tinea unguium—more proximal involvement of the great toenails than in Figure 3.2.
The great toenail on the left is totally dystrophic.

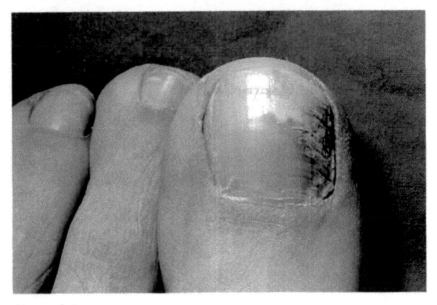

Figure 3.4
Tinea unguium—superficial 'white' type.

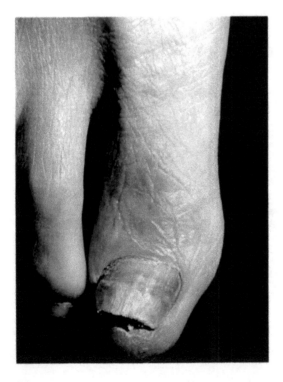

Figure 3.5
Tinea unguium—yellow discoloration with fragility of the nail plate developing.

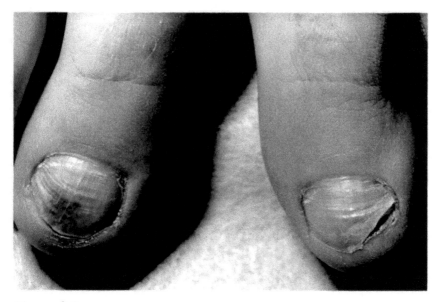

Figure 3.6
Tinea unguium—secondary to trauma in a long-distance runner.

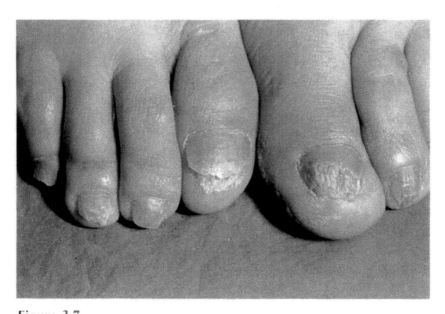

Figure 3.7
Tinea unguium—late stage, showing considerable thickening.

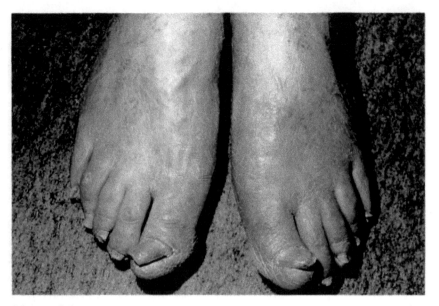

Figure 3.8
Tinea unguium—late stage with onychogryphosis.

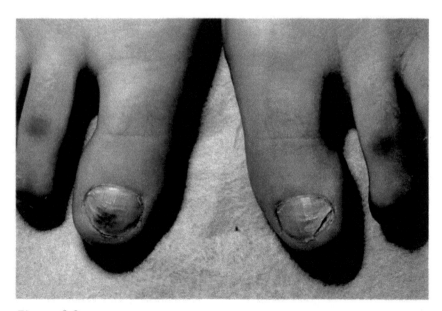

Figure 3.9
Tinea unguium colonized by the saprophytic fungus S. brevicaulis. This type of colonization may occur in the nails of long-distance runners.

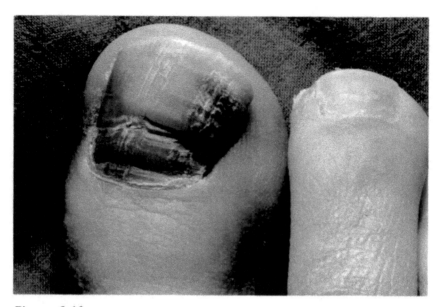

Figure 3.10
Tinea unguium (as in Figure 3.9)—a later stage.

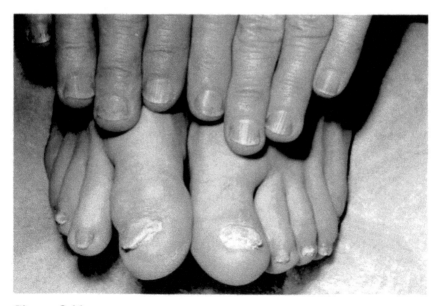

Figure 3.11
Tinea unguium—hand and foot involvement.

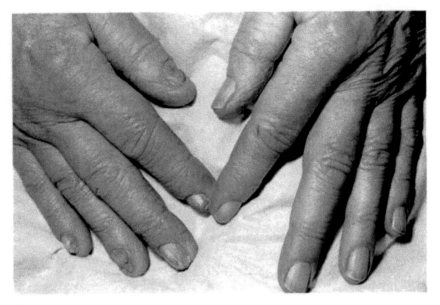

Figure 3.12
Tinea unguium—right hand only involved.

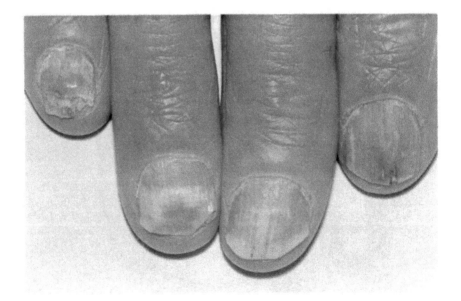

Figure 3.13
Tinea unguium—four nails on the right hand are involved. There is a varying degree of proximal spread in the different digits.

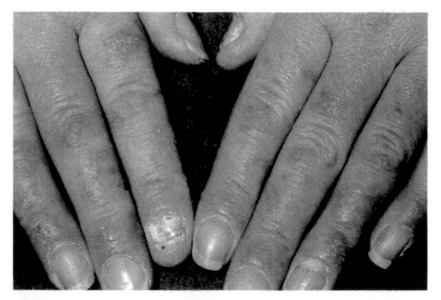

Figure 3.14
Tinea unguium—severe dystrophy of the right index fingernail only.

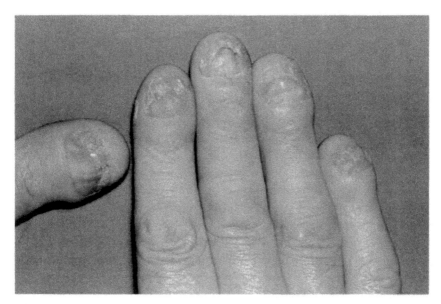

Figure 3.15
Tinea unguium—severe dystrophy of all the digits.

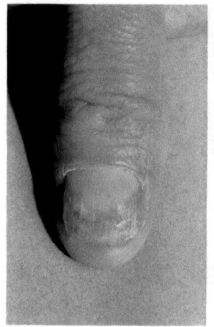

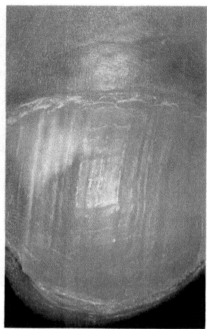

Figure 3.16
Tinea unguium—an onycholytic type with nail-plate fragility.

Figure 3.17
Proximal subungual onychomycosis.

(total 'dystrophic' onychomycosis) as a result of fungal invasion is relatively rare, and it usually takes several years to reach this stage.

Distal-lateral subungual onychomycosis (DLSO) is typically caused by *Trichophyton rubrum* and, less commonly, by *T. mentagrophytes* var. *interdigitale*. Other dermatophytes are rarely responsible. DLSO may be limited to the toenails, but fingernails may sometimes be affected, an infection which presents as the 'one hand—two feet' syndrome. When DLSO involves the fingernails, palmar infection with scaling is usually present. Infection of the inguinal folds may also be observed. *Trichophyton rubrum* var. *nigricans* ('melanoid' strain) onychomycosis occasionally produces a black pigmentation of the nail as a result of the direct production of melanin-related pigment by the fungus.

In proximal subungual onychomycosis (PSO), dermatophytes breach the nail matrix keratogenous zone through the proximal nail-fold horny layer. Fungal elements are then found in the ventral nail but these provoke little

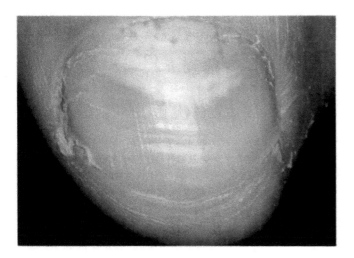

Figure 3.18
Proximal subungual onychomycosis.

Figure 3.19
White superficial onychomycosis.

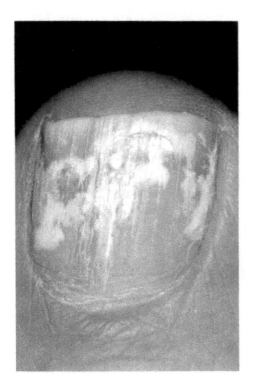

inflammatory reaction. PSO presents as an area of whiteness in the proximal portion of the nail plate. The nail-plate surface is normal because the fungi do not penetrate the dorsal nail. This type of onychomycosis was very rare before the advent of HIV and AIDS. In recent years, however, it has become common in AIDS patients, in whom it often affects several digits simultaneously.

In white superficial onychomycosis (WSO), the dermatophytes invade the most superficial layers of the nail plate but do not penetrate it. The nail surface displays small, white, opaque, friable spots that are a manifestation of the fungal colonies present in the most superficial layers of the nail plate; the whole nail may ultimately be infected. WSO is almost always caused by *T. mentagrophytes* var. *interdigitale* and is associated with concurrent tinea pedis interdigitalis. Invasion of the superficial nail plate by *T. rubrum* var. *nigricans* (as well as the non-dermatophytic mould *Scytalydium dimidiatum*) is the cause of the so-called 'black superficial onychomycosis', in which the nail-plate surface displays pigmented spots.

In endonyx onychomycosis (EO), the dermatophytes reach the nail plate through the plantar skin (as in DLSO) (Figure 3.20). However, rather than

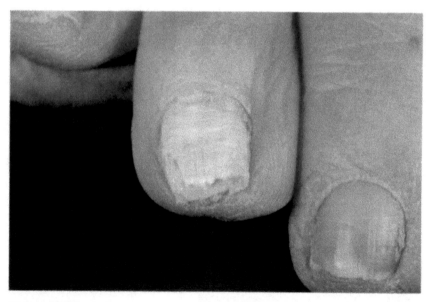

Figure 3.20
In endonyx onychomycosis, dermatophytes invade and penetrate the whole thickness of the nail plate. In this case the causative agent is T. rubrum, *although most often* T. soudanense *is responsible.*

colonising the nail bed, fungal elements immediately invade and penetrate the nail plate. This variety of onychomycosis is frequently associated with *T. soudanense* infection. EO produces a milky-white discoloration of the nail plate without subungual thickening and onycholysis. Plantar infection is usually present.

Total dystrophic onychomycosis is the most advanced form of all these types of infection. In such cases, the whole nail bed and overlying nail plate are uniformly invaded.

The diagnosis of dermatophyte nail invasion can be established by isolating and identifying the fungi from the affected nail provided the patient has not recently (2–3 months) taken a local or systemic antifungal agent. The exact site from which diagnostic specimens should be taken depends entirely on the type of onychomycosis:

- In DLSO, subungual tissue should be collected from the nail bed after the overlying onycholytic nail plate has been clipped away. It is very important to obtain material from the most proximal portion of the affected nail bed since more distal areas of the dystrophy may contain only non-viable fungus.
- In PSO, the fungi are only in the ventral nail plate. When the affected area is very proximal to the distal edge of the nail, the collection of specimens requires punch biopsy of the nail plate.
- In WSO, the material can be easily obtained by scraping the white or black areas on the superficial nail plate.
- In EO, distal nail clippings contain many fungal elements and these can be used directly for culture.

Direct microscopic examination of the specimens can be performed using KOH preparations. Nail or nail-bed debris is placed on a glass slide and a drop of 40% KOH solution with ink (3 ml of KOH solution mixed with one cartridge of ink) is added. After the cover-slip has been put in place, the slide is placed in a moist chamber for 2 hours to allow the keratin to clear. It is then viewed under a microscope. A formulation of KOH and dimethylsulphoxide (DMSO) makes for faster clearing of the specimens (see Chapter 1).

Cultures are most commonly performed using Sabouraud's medium with 0.05% chloramphenicol and 0.4% cycloheximide (actidione). These are incubated at 26–28 °C for 2–3 weeks. Gross colony morphology and microscopic examination of the mycelia stained with lactophenol cotton blue permit the identification of the commonest causative dermatophytes.

The isolation of dermatophytes from the nails may be difficult as the fungi may be scarcely viable and will not grow in cultures. The failure rate for nail culture is high (20–30%), and cultures should always be repeated when the clinical picture strongly suggests onychomycosis. Examination of material taken from associated skin lesions is advisable since these usually demonstrate profuse dermatophyte growth. If a skin culture proves positive, nail cultures should be repeated and a nail-plate biopsy considered, if necessary. A formal biopsy, as for any other disease, may eventually be required if the differential diagnosis cannot be resolved by other means. Prior to this, any thickened nail that is thought to be fungal can be clipped off and submitted for routine biopsy procedures. Fungal stains (e.g. PAS) exhibit any fungal elements as a clear red (Figure 3.21).

Differential diagnosis

The differential diagnosis between onychomycosis and many types of psoriatic nail dystrophy can be very difficult, since subungual hyperkeratosis, onycholysis, splinter haemorrhage and diffuse nail 'crumbling' are clinical signs of both conditions (Figure 3.22). Dermatophytes or other fungi can also sometimes colonise psoriatic nails, particularly when the nail plate is grossly deformed—a positive culture does not exclude the diagnosis of psoriasis! Some other conditions that may mimic onychomycosis are shown in Figures 3.23–3.44.

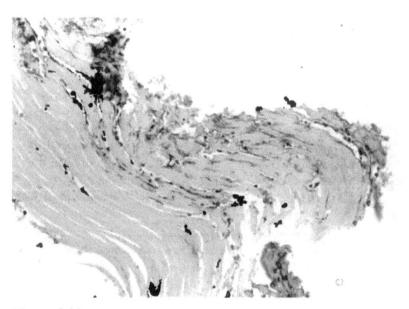

Figure 3.21
A section of a nail stained with PAS to show all the fungal components present. The section was taken from thickened nail tissue which was removed with chiropody clippers, fixed in formalin and processed as in any biopsy (Scher technique).

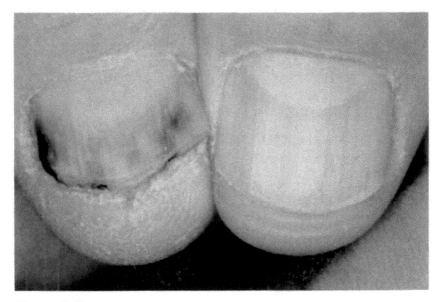

Figure 3.22

Tinea unguium in right thumbnail. The black colour under the nail plate is oily dirt.

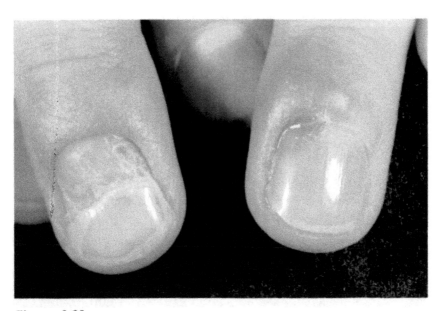

Figure 3.23

Tinea unguium—differential diagnosis: acute paronychia.

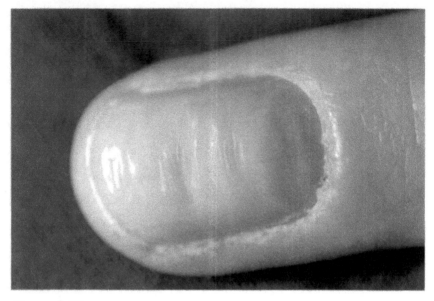

Figure 3.24
Tinea unguium—differential diagnosis: chronic paronychia.

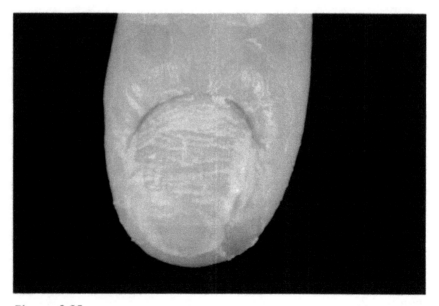

Figure 3.25
Tinea unguium—differential diagnosis: chronic paronychia.

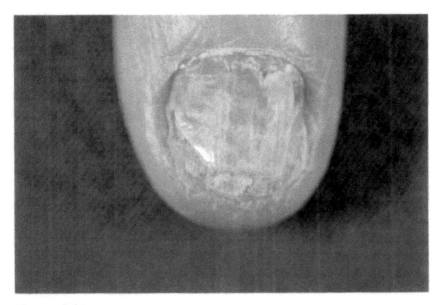

Figure 3.26
Tinea unguium—differential diagnosis: chronic eczema.

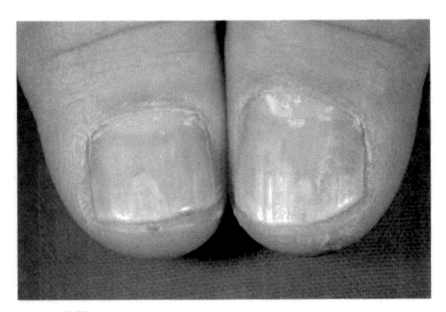

Figure 3.27
Tinea unguium—differential diagnosis: psoriatic fingernail.

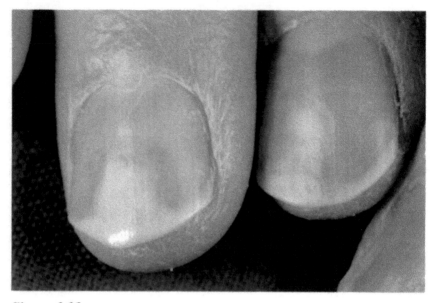

Figure 3.28
Tinea unguium—differential diagnosis: psoriatic fingernail.

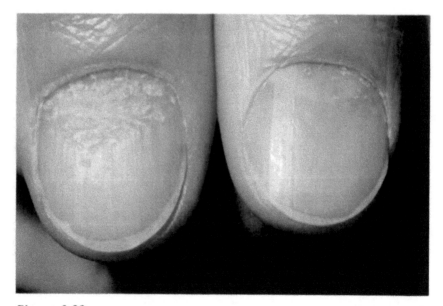

Figure 3.29
Tinea unguium—differential diagnosis: psoriatic fingernail.

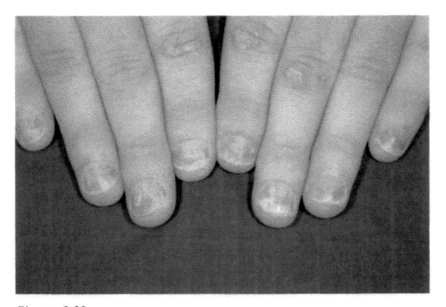

Figure 3.30
Tinea unguium—differential diagnosis: psoriatic fingernail.

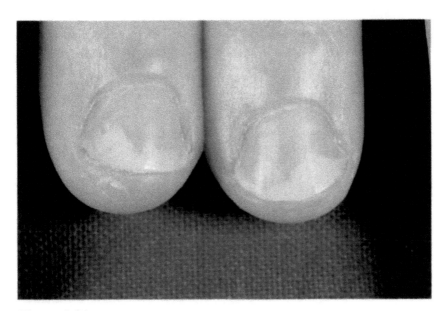

Figure 3.31
Tinea unguium—differential diagnosis: psoriatic fingernail.

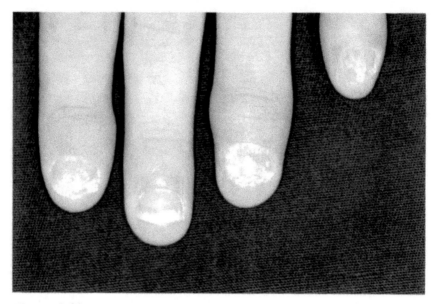

Figure 3.32
Tinea unguium—differential diagnosis: acrodermatitis continua.

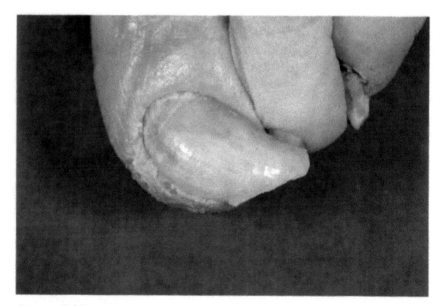

Figure 3.33
Tinea unguium—differential diagnosis: onychogryphosis.

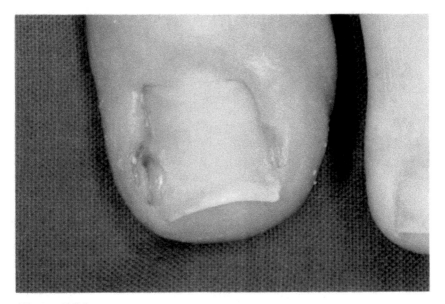

Figure 3.34
Tinea unguium—differential diagnosis: an ingrown toenail.

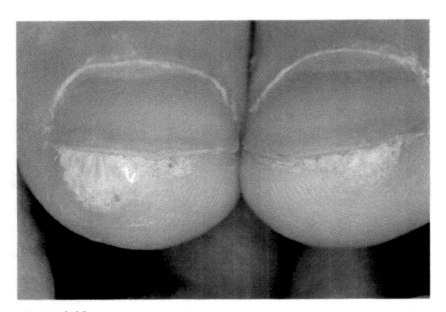

Figure 3.35
Tinea unguium—differential diagnosis: subungual warts.

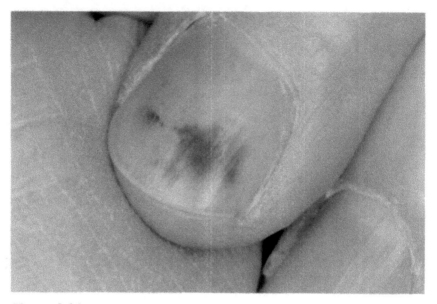

Figure 3.36
Tinea unguium—differential diagnosis: hematoma.

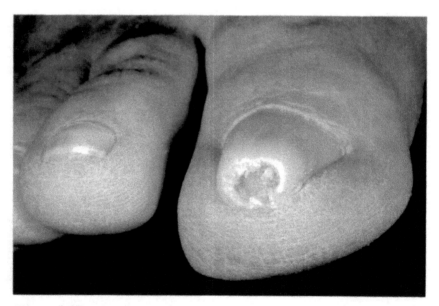

Figure 3.37
Tinea unguium—differential diagnosis: trumpet nail.

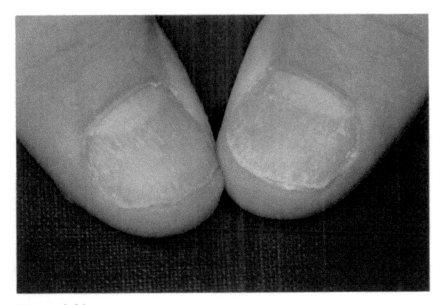

Figure 3.38
Tinea unguium—differential diagnosis: trachyonychia ('rough' nail).

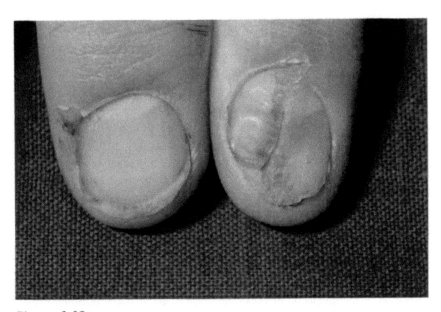

Figure 3.39
Tinea unguium—differential diagnosis: trauma (knife damage in youth).

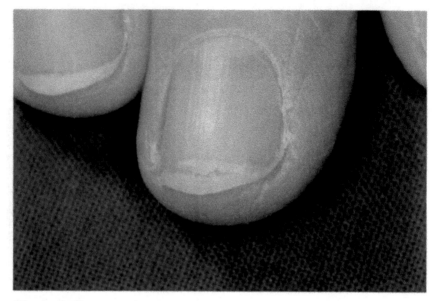

Figure 3.40
Tinea unguium—differential diagnosis: onychoschizia ('layering' of the nail).

Onychomycosis due to non-dermatophytic moulds

Moulds that have been proven to cause onychomycosis (see Chapter 1) include *Scytalydium* species (*Hendersonula toruloidea*), *Scopulariopsis brevicaulis* and *Fusarium* species. The latter may produce DLSO, WSO and PSO with paronychia. *Scytalydium* species and *Scopulariopsis* produce nail lesions indistinguishable from DLSO. At its most distinctive, the latter produces infected areas that are prominently creamy-yellow in colour. *Scytalydium dimidiatum* may also produce black, superficial onychomycosis. Even though moulds may be isolated from dystrophic toenails, their role as primary pathogens is still unclear as they most commonly colonise nails with pre-existing nail disease—typically, dermatophytic onychomycosis or traumatic dystrophies.

The diagnosis of non-dermatophytic mould nail infection requires the isolation of the fungus on direct examination of the material obtained from the suspected lesion; and repeated isolation by culture of a species of fungus consistent with the finding on direct microscopic examination. Cultures for dermatophytes should also be regularly negative.

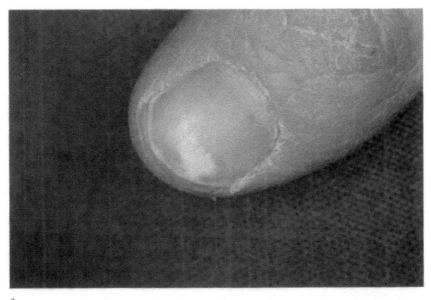

a

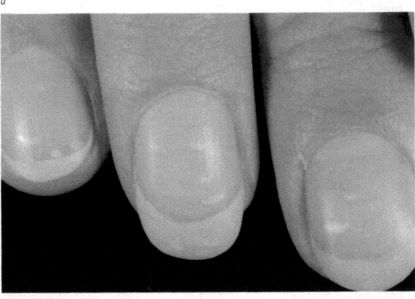

b

Figure 3.41
Tinea unguium—differential diagnosis: 'white spots' (a and b).

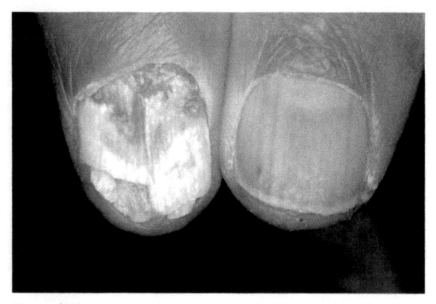

Figure 3.42
Tinea unguium—differential diagnosis: a post-traumatic dystrophy. Saprophytic growth only.

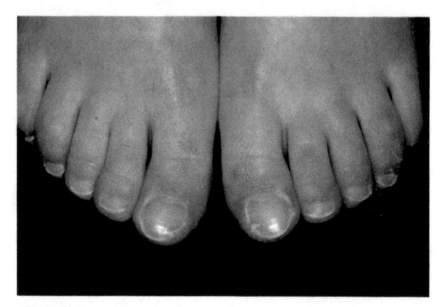

Figure 3.43
Tinea unguium—differential diagnosis: shoe trauma on the long big toenail.

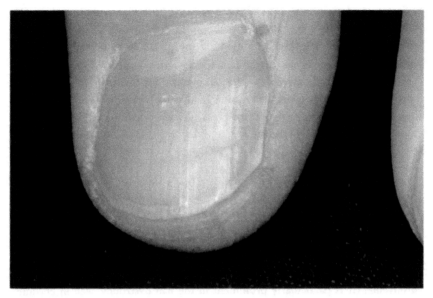

Figure 3.44
Tinea unguium—differential diagnosis: onycholysis of unknown aetiology, recurrent; eventual spontaneous cure.

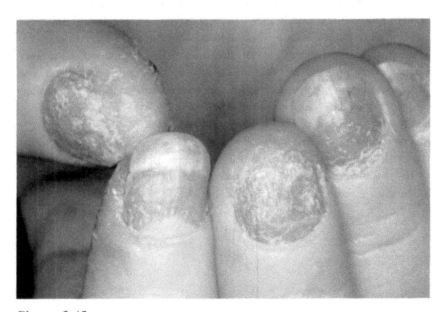

Figure 3.45
Candida infection—chronic mucocutaneous candidiasis (CMC).

Since non-dermatophytic moulds are sensitive to cycloheximide and do not grow on any medium containing this antibiotic, Sabouraud's dextrose agar without cycloheximide should be used for any specimen suspected of containing these pathogens. *Scytalydium* species grow in up to 3 days at 26 °C.

This type of onychomycosis is rare, accounting for less than 3% of nail fungal infections. It is generally considered that such organisms are secondary to primary traumatic or other dystrophies. Because of this, significant colonisations are usually treated.

Candida onychomycosis

Primary nail-plate invasion by *Candida albicans* is extremely rare in the absence of immunosuppression. However, *C. albicans* commonly grows from the subungual area in onycholytic nails and from the proximal nail fold in chronic paronychia. (It is particularly prominent in the nail dystrophy seen in chronic mucocutaneous candidiasis Figure 3.45.)

C. albicans can frequently be isolated from the subungual area of onycholytic nails as well as from the proximal nail fold in chronic paronychia. However, in both these conditions, *Candida* colonisation is a secondary phenomenon since topical or systemic antimycotics do not cure the nail abnormalities. Nail invasion by *C. albicans* usually indicates an underlying immunological defect and is most frequently seen in chronic mucocutaneous candidiasis; in the latter, *C. albicans* invasion of the nail plate is associated with an inflammatory reaction of the proximal nail fold, nail matrix, nail bed and hyponychium. The affected digits have a terminal swollen appearance, with erythema and swelling of the proximal and lateral nail folds. The nail bed is hyperkeratotic and the nail plate is thickened and highly dystrophic as a result of diffuse 'fragmentation'. Complete disruption of the nail plate is almost always observed. Oral candidiasis is present in the majority of affected individuals.

The diagnosis of *Candida* nail invasion is made by culturing nail scrapings in Sabouraud's medium at 37 °C (see Chapter 1).

4 THERAPY FOR SKIN, HAIR AND NAIL FUNGAL INFECTIONS

The relatively recent development of successful antifungal drugs has revolutionized the clinician's attitude to, and management of, fungal infection or colonization. Such drugs assume even more importance now that the wider use of immunosuppressive drugs can induce more severe forms of fungal 'invasion'. In AIDS, for example, usually innocuous 'commensals' may now be detected in the internal organs.

Most of the fungi that affect the skin, hair and nails only proliferate under the ideal conditions of warmth, moisture and humidity. Male skin is also more 'attractive' to dermatophytes. Hence non-specific actions and treatments may, under certain circumstances, be as important as specific drug regimens. For example:

*   minimising the risk of trauma to the nails;
*   minimising trauma and softening of the periungual tissues when employed in occupations that involve frequent contact with water;
*   maintaining dryness in the body folds, in particular the:
    *   interdigital spaces of the feet
    *   groin
    *   axillae
    *   submammary
        folds of adipose tissue; and
*   attending promptly to orthopaedic and podiatric problems.

It is important to treat symptomatic tinea pedis and onychomycosis. Untreated tinea pedis may lead to severe reactive inflammation, with painful fissuring of the feet and toes. Occasionally, generalized 'autosensitisation' eruptions occur in response to persistent focal fungal skin disease. Onychomycosis may be asymptomatic and no more than an 'aesthetic compromise' in its early stages. However, progression of the disease frequently leads to complications, such as an ingrowing toenail and sometimes the painful nail-plate deformities of onychogryphosis and pincer or trumpet nail that may occur later in life. Studies of onychogryphosis in the elderly have shown that many such patients had untreated onychomycosis at a younger age. The initial capital cost of treating onychomycosis successfully is, therefore, fully justified.

On the foot, the treatment principles involve the removal of the site of infection (the stratum corneum) with keratolytics and the use of specific antifungal drugs. Surgical methods will rarely be involved.

Keratolytics may be used alone or in combination with drying or antifungal powders; oral therapy may be used if the infection is severe. The most common keratolytic is salicylic acid—e.g. 3% salicylic acid and 6% benzoic acid (Whitfield's ointment).

Specific antifungal compounds include the following:

- Azole drugs, such as imidazoles and triazoles, e.g. miconazole, econazole, ketoconazole, itraconazole, tioconazole and fluconazole.
- Allylamines, e.g. terbinafine and naftifine.
- A miscellaneous group that includes griseofulvin (oral), tolnaftate, amorolfine and cyclopiroxolamine.

Most antifungal drugs are fungistatic at therapeutic concentrations. Terbinafine (topical and oral) is fungicidal against dermatophytes and some yeasts and non-dermatophyte moulds. Due to this and because of the fact that terbinafine enters the skin and nail tissues very rapidly where it is maintained, terbinafine can be used for very short periods with high efficacy. According to several double-blind clinical studies comparing both topical and oral terbinafine with other antimycotics, terbinafine was shown to be more efficacious.

Topical therapy

Topical therapy may be sufficient for dermatophytosis other than nail and scalp infections—for example, terbinafine topical formulations, tolnaftate, imidazole, amorolfine, cyclopiroxolamine, clotrimazole, miconazole, econazole, ketoconazole, bifonazole and tioconazole. Terbinafine, which has the shortest treatment time of topical antifungals, takes about one week to kill the fungus but the skin will take about 2–4 weeks to return to normal.

Inorganic agents (such as selenium sulphide shampoo) are widely used for pityrosporum yeast infection, particularly for pityriasis capitis and mild forms of pityriasis (tinea) versicolor. The most appropriate antifungal treatment for pityriasis versicolor is to use a topical imidazole or terbinafine, in a solution or lathering preparation. Ketoconazole shampoo has been proven to be very effective. Alternative treatments include zinc pyrithione or selenium sulfide shampoo applied daily for 10–14 days, or the use of propylene glycol 50% in water twice daily for 14 days. In severe cases with extensive lesions, or in cases with lesions resistant to topical treatment or in cases of frequent relapse, oral therapy is usually effective. Mycologically, yeast cells may still be seen in skin scrapings for up to 30 days following treatment. Patients should thus be monitored on clinical grounds. Patients also need to be warned that it may take many months for their skin pigmentation to return to normal, even after the infection has been successfully treated. Relapse is a regular occurrence, and prophylactic treatment with a topical agent once weekly is often necessary to avoid recurrence.

Most cases of Pityrosporum folliculitis respond well to topical imidazole treatment. However, patients with extensive lesions often require oral treatment with ketoconazole or itraconazole. Once again, prophylactic treatment once or twice a week is mandatory to prevent relapse, which is unfortunately common.

The only topical agents that have some success in combating nail infection are amorolfine, cyclopiroxolamine and tioconazole. These agents alone may be successful in treating mild or childhood onychomycosis, and it is reasonable to use this modality first in children in view of the established side-effect profile of all the known systemic antifungal agents. It has also been suggested, but not proven, that these may be valuable as prophylaxis against onychomycosis in immunosuppressed individuals. In these cases the infection is often severe and may preface systemic spread.

Tinea capitis always requires oral therapy.

Oral therapy

The oral agents against fungi have revolutionised the clinical management of severe and symptomatic infections. However, in onychomycosis, 'cure' is evidently not 100%. In skin and nail infections, cure rates are now sufficiently good that failure of treatment suggests one should think that the fungal growth was not the *prime* cause. If the affected nail is sufficiently dystrophic and thickened, then urea avulsion may be useful. This enables the affected nail to be removed. Urea paste (40%) is applied under occlusion for 1 week before cutting away the affected nail (Figure 4.1).

In symptomatic onychomycosis, tinea capitis and in systemic fungal infections associated with immunosuppression, oral therapy is the treatment of choice. Table 4.1 outlines some of the dose regimes recommended for the commonest infections seen in routine clinical practice.

Table 4.1 Oral treatment options for cutaneous fungal infections

Infection	Treatment options
Tinea unguium (Onychomycosis)	Terbinafine 250 mg/day for 6 weeks for fingernails, 12 weeks for toenails Itraconazole 200 mg/day for 3–5 months or 400 mg/day for 1 week per month for 3–4 consecutive months Fluconazole 150–300 mg/week until cured (~30 weeks) Griseofulvin 500–1000 mg/day until cured (~12–18 months)
Tinea capitis	Griseofulvin 500 mg/day (not less than 10 mg/kg/day) until cured (up to 12 weeks) Terbinafine 250 mg/day for 4 weeks Itraconazole 100 mg/day for 4 weeks Fluconazole 100 mg/day for 4 weeks
Tinea corporis	Terbinafine 250 mg/day for 2 weeks Itraconazole 100 mg/day for 15 days or 200 mg/day for 1 week Fluconazole 150–300 mg/week for 4 weeks Griseofulvin 500 mg/day until cured (4–6 weeks), often combined with a topical imidazole agent
Tinea cruris	Terbinafine 250 mg/day for 2 weeks Itraconazole 100 mg/day for 15 days or 200 mg/day for 1 week Fluconazole 150–300 mg/week for 4 weeks Griseofulvin 500 mg/day until cured (4–6 weeks)
Tinea pedis	Terbinafine 250 mg/day for 2–4 weeks Itraconazole 100 mg/day for 4 weeks Fluconazole 150–300 mg/week for 4 weeks Griseofulvin 500 mg/day until cured (4–6 weeks)
Chronic and/or widespread non-responsive tinea	Terbinafine 250 mg/day for 4–6 weeks Itraconazole 200 mg/day for 4–6 weeks Griseofulvin 500–1000 mg/day until cured (3–6 months)
Chronic or severe non-responsive pityriasis versicolor or pityriasis capitis	Itraconazole 200 mg/day for 1 week Fluconazole 150 mg/week for 4 weeks Ketoconazole 400 mg single dose or 200 mg/day for 5–10 days
Chronic/recurrent mucocutaneous candidiasis	Fluconazole 150 mg/week for 4 weeks Itraconazole 200 mg/day for 1 week Ketoconazole 200 mg/day for 5–10 days

Vaginal candidiasis	Fluconazole 150 mg single dose
	Itraconazole 400 mg single dose (two 200 mg doses 8 hours apart)
Candidiasis of the nail	Itraconazole 200 mg/day for 3–5 months or 400 mg/day for 1 week per month for 3–4 consecutive months
	Fluconazole 150–300 mg/week until cured (~30 weeks)

Note:
Consult the relevant product information sheet for prescribing details.

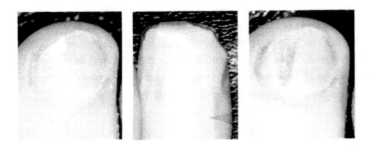

Figure 4.1

Urea paste nail avulsion. Most of the affected nail is easily removed after 1 week of paste application. (Courtesy of Dr R Baran, Cannes, France.)

Griseofulvin

Griseofulvin is an oral fungistatic agent derived from a number of *Penicillium* species. It binds to microtubular proteins and inhibits both dermatophyte cell division and nucleic acid synthesis. It has been available for over 30 years and is still valuable for dermatophytic skin infection, in particular tinea capitis. Oral therapy using griseofulvin has been used extensively for the treatment of dermatophytosis (tinea or ringworm). However, it is ineffective against cutaneous candidiasis, pityriasis versicolor and moulds. The usual adult dose is 500 mg to 1 gm/day; an ultramicrosize formulation of 330 mg/day is also available (not less than 10 mg/kg should be given). However, higher doses of 1000 mg/day are commonly given when treating nail infections. The dose for children under 25 kg is 10 mg/kg and 250–500 mg for children over 25 kg. The duration of therapy varies from patient to patient and on the site and severity of the infection, with up to 12 weeks being required for skin and hair infections and approximately 12 months for nails. Relapse is common, especially for nails, where between 40 and 70% of patients fail treatment.

119

Griseofulvin is usually well tolerated although it is best taken with food, which also facilitates absorption. It accumulates in the stratum corneum within 4–6 hours after administration. However, it has a low affinity for keratin, and drug levels in keratin decline rapidly within 48–72 hours after discontinuation of therapy. This lack of binding with keratin may explain why griseofulvin has such a low cure rate (20–30%) in toenail infections. Adverse effects include headache, gastrointestinal disturbance and, less commonly, urticaria, diarrhoea and photosensitivity. The drug should be avoided during pregnancy and in patients with liver disease. Griseofulvin can diminish the anticoagulant effect of warfarin and concurrent administration of phenobarbitone may interfere with absorption. It may also interact with alcohol, causing a disulfiram-type reaction. Patients should thus avoid alcohol. Resistance to griseofulvin is rarely reported and treatment failure is usually due to other factors, such as poor absorption, poor nail-tissue concentrations or insufficient treatment duration. Griseofulvin was the first oral antifungal agent effective against dermatophytes. It is relatively free of serious adverse effects but requires long treatment times. Relapse rates are high.

Ketoconazole

Ketoconazole is an oral or topical synthetic dioxolane imidazole compound that interferes with the biosynthesis of ergosterol. This leads to alterations in a number of membrane-associated cell functions. It has a broad spectrum of activity that includes both dermatophytes and yeasts. It was the first available orally active imidazole. Ketoconazole is not absorbed after topical application but it is well absorbed orally under acid conditions. It is poorly absorbed in patients with achlorhydria and in those taking antacids or H_2-receptor antagonists. The usual adult dose is 200–400 mg/day depending on the infection. When required for children, a dose of 3 mg/kg can be used. The duration of treatment will depend on the nature of the infection. However, liver function must be monitored in patients receiving treatment for more than 30 days. The most common side-effects are nausea, anorexia and vomiting, which occur in about 20% of patients. Adrenal or testicular steroid metabolism may be affected. The coadministration of terfenadine, astemizole or cisapride is potentially fatal and should hence be avoided. Ketoconazole also enhances the effects of warfarin, oral hypoglycaemics and phenytoin. Oral ketoconazole has a high affinity for keratin and it has been used for dermatophytes, although the risk of hepatitis, albeit rare, makes this a secondary choice for therapy, especially now newer agents such as fluconazole, itraconazole and terbinafine are available. Ketoconazole remains, however, as an important adjunct in the treatment of AIDS patients with fluconazole-resistant *Candida* infections.

Fluconazole

Fluconazole is an oral synthetic bis-triazole compound that inhibits the cytochrome P450–dependent 14 alpha-demethylation step in the formation of ergosterol, which leads to alterations in a number of membrane-associated cell functions. Fluconazole has a broad spectrum of activity that includes both dermatophytes and yeasts. It is water soluble and is rapidly absorbed, with good penetration into all tissues and body fluids. Absorption is not dependent on acid conditions and is also unaffected by food intake. Unlike other azoles, fluconazole is not metabolised in humans and it is largely excreted unchanged in the urine. The usual adult doses range between 100 and 400 mg/day, depending on the immune status of the patient, the infecting organism and the patient's response to therapy. With most mucocutaneous diseases, it is usual to start with a higher dose of 400 mg/day for the first two days and then reduce to 100–200 mg/day. Vaginal candidiasis usually responds to a single dose of 150 mg. Fluconazole is generally well tolerated. It has minor side-effects, such as nausea and vomiting, which occur in a few patients. Unlike ketoconazole and itraconazole, fluconazole has few significant drug interactions. However, the effects of warfarin, cyclosporin A, oral hypoglycaemics, phenytoin, midazolam and theophylline may be increased by fluconazole when given in doses of 200 mg/day or higher. Fluconazole has been proven to be particularly effective in the treatment of mucosal and cutaneous forms of candidiasis. It is currently the drug of choice for controlling oropharyngeal candidiasis in AIDS patients.

Itraconazole

Itraconazole is an oral fungistatic synthetic dioxolane triazole compound that inhibits the cytochrome P450-dependent 14 alpha-demethylation step in the formation of ergosterol, which leads to alterations in a number of membrane-associated cell functions. It has a broad spectrum of activity that includes dermatophytes, yeasts and some moulds. Itraconazole is insoluble in aqueous solvents and its absorption from the gastrointestinal tract is often incomplete (about 55%). However, absorption is improved if the drug is given with food or under acid conditions. Itraconazole is more than 99% protein bound in serum, which produces low plasma and cerebrospinal (CSF) levels. However, it is extensively distributed into lipophilic tissues and accumulates in the liver, brain and skin. Itraconazole is degraded in the liver into a large number of metabolites that are excreted with bile and urine. The usual adult dose for cutaneous infections is 100–400 mg/day, depending on the infection. Itraconazole is generally well tolerated and it has minor side-effects, nausea, headache and abdominal pain being reported in a few patients. Unlike ketoconazole it does not affect adrenal or testicular steroid metabolism. Itraconazole concentrations are reduced following concomitant administration of phenytoin, rifampicin, antacids and H_2-antagonists. Coadministration of terfenadine, cisapride or astemizole with itraconazole is contraindicated, and the effects of warfarin, oral hypoglycaemics, phenytoin, digoxin, midazolam, triazolam, calcium antagonists (of dihydropyridine type), chinidin, cyclosporin-A, tacrolimus and methyl prednisolone are enhanced. Itraconazole can be used to treat various cutaneous infections, including dermatophytosis, onychomycosis, pityriasis versicolor and oral and vaginal forms of candidiasis. Systemic ketoconazole that preceded itraconazole was to some degree hepatotoxic; this is much less common with itraconazole, although still possible.

Terbinafine

Terbinafine is an oral or topical synthetic allylamine compound that inhibits the action of squalene epoxidase, a crucial enzyme in the formation of ergosterol. This leads to membrane disruption and cell death. It is important to note that it is fungicidal against dermatophytes such as *Trichophyton*, *Microsporum* and *Epidermiphyton floccosum* species. It is also effective against moulds, dimorphic fungi and many yeasts of the genera *Pityrosporum*, *Candida* and *Rhodoturula*. The antimycotic activity of terbinafine is a consequence of its interference with ergosterol biosynthesis, especially its inhibition of fungal squalene epoxidase: squalene accumulates within the cell, which leads to concentrations that are toxic to the fungal cell. The drug is well absorbed after oral administration and is strongly lipophilic, being concentrated in the dermis, epidermis and adipose tissue. It has been detected in the distal portion of nails after 4 weeks of treatment, indicating that diffusion from the nail bed is a major factor in drug penetration. Terbinafine is metabolised by the liver and the inactive metabolites are excreted in the urine. The usual adult dose is 250 mg/day, with the duration of treatment being dependent on the site and extent of the infection. This can range from 2 weeks for interdigital tinea pedis, 4–6 weeks for widespread or chronic non-responsive dermatophytosis of skin and/or scalp, to 12 weeks for toenails (Figures 4.2–4.4). Terbinafine is generally well tolerated. The commonest side-effects are nausea, abdominal pain and allergic skin reactions, but these are often mild and transient. Transient taste disturbances are occasionally reported. Oral terbinafine has become an important drug, particularly for dermatophytosis of the nail. It can also be used to treat dermatophytosis of the skin and/or scalp.

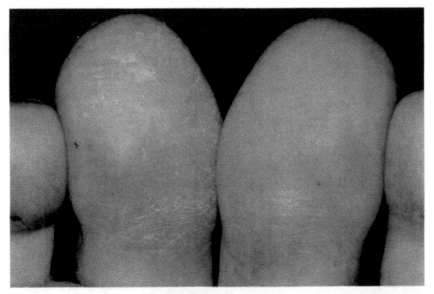

a

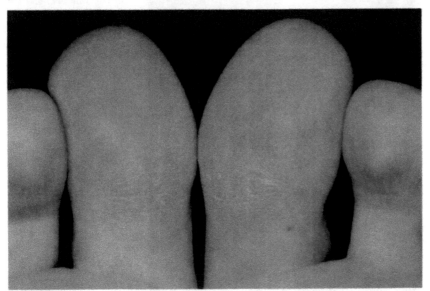

b

Figure 4.2

(a) 'Dry-type' plantar tinea is almost without exception caused by the dermatophyte
Trichophyton rubrum. *It is characterised by minor scales, as remnants of very*
superficial vesicles. In spite of fairly mild symptoms, this form of dermatophytosis is best
treated with oral antifungals for a long period of remission, or even permanent cure.
(b) A two-week course of oral terbinafine at a dose of 250 mg once daily resulted in
complete cure.

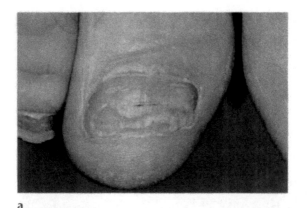

a

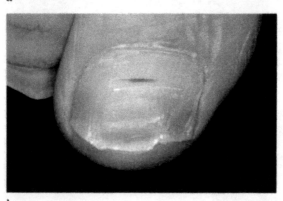

b

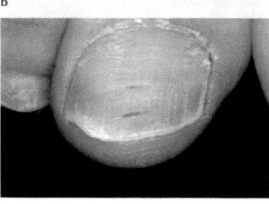

c

Figure 4.3
(a) Onychomycosis in the large toenail, caused by the dermatophyte T. rubrum. The nail was treated with a course of oral terbinafine at a dose of 250 mg once daily for 12 weeks. (b) The result one year after the beginning of treatment. There is no sign of fungal disease, but there is residual deformation of the nail plate. (c) The result one and a half years after the start of treatment. There is no sign of infection, and the contour of the nail plate is normal as well.

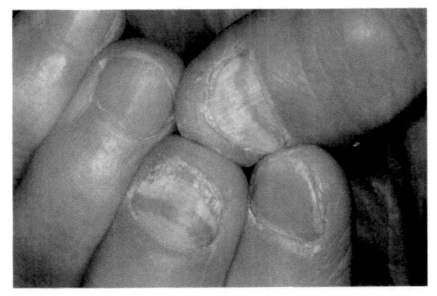

a

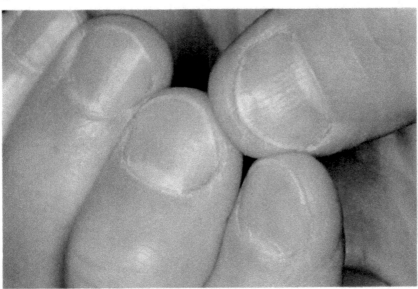

b

Figure 4.4

(a) Onychomycosis in the fingernails, caused by the dermatophyte T. rubrum. *Typically, the skin of these fingers shows fine scales. Oral terbinafine was administered at a dose of 250 mg once daily for 8 weeks. (b) Four months later, the skin and nails are cured.*

INDEX

Page references in **bold** refer to figures; those in *italic* refer to tables.